The
COMPLETE
LOW
LECTIN
Food List Guide

Essential Foods and Recipes

Transform Your Diet and Well-being with Our Complete Ingredient List and Meal Ideas

CAROLINE SANDFORD, BSN RN

TABLE OF CONTENTS

To David, my greatest strength and support.

To my sons, Isaac and Eli, my true source of inspiration,

And to all my patients, whom I consider my friends;

This book would not have been made possible if not for all of you.

- Caroline -

Chapter 1: Introduction

Welcome to the Guide

Welcome to The Complete Low Lectin Food List Guide! If you're reading this, you may be seeking to improve your health through dietary changes or are simply curious about the low lectin diet. This guide is designed to provide you with comprehensive information about lectins, their impact on health, and how you can successfully incorporate a low lectin diet into your life.

Lectins are proteins found in many foods, particularly in legumes, grains, and certain vegetables. For some individuals, high lectin consumption can lead to digestive issues and inflammation. This guide aims to simplify the complexities surrounding lectins and empower you to make informed dietary choices that can enhance your well-being.

Author's Journey: Caroline Sandford's Story

I'm Caroline Sandford, a dedicated nurse and health advocate with nearly two decades of experience in immunology, focusing on adult endocrinology. My journey into the world of nutrition and dietary interventions began when I recognized the profound impact that food choices can have on health outcomes. As a second-generation Filipino immigrant, my passion for health has been shaped by my cultural background and personal experiences, particularly as a mother to two teenage boys.

My exploration of low lectin diets was sparked by witnessing the positive changes in my patients who adopted dietary modifications to manage chronic conditions. I realized that many individuals were overwhelmed by the conflicting information surrounding dietary guidelines, particularly regarding lectins. This led me to create this guide, which combines my nursing expertise with a passion for nutrition to provide clear, actionable advice.

Through my personal and professional experiences, I have become a strong advocate for the benefits of eliminating high lectin foods from one's diet. My goal is to make the journey of adopting a low lectin lifestyle accessible and enjoyable, empowering you to take charge of your health.

Chapter 2: Scientific Research Advancements

Not long ago, I met Daniel, a 45-year-old father of two who had been struggling with fatigue, digestive issues, and joint pain for years. After extensive research and consultations with various nutritionists, he discovered the concept of a low lectin diet. With a mix of skepticism and hope, Daniel decided to eliminate high lectin foods—like certain legumes, whole grains, and nightshade vegetables—from his diet. To his surprise, within just a few weeks, he felt more energetic, his digestive issues subsided, and his joint pain began to diminish. Daniel's experience is a testament to the potential benefits of understanding and managing lectin intake for individuals of all ages.

Recent Findings on Lectins and Health

Recent research has illuminated the complex role that lectins play in human health. Lectins are proteins found in a variety of foods, particularly in beans, legumes, grains, and some vegetables. While they serve a protective function in plants, they can bind to carbohydrates in the human gut, potentially leading to digestive disturbances and inflammation. A study published in the **Journal of Nutritional Biochemistry** highlighted that high lectin consumption is associated with increased gastrointestinal symptoms and may exacerbate conditions like leaky gut syndrome (Liu et al., 2021).

Moreover, cooking methods can significantly reduce the lectin content in foods. For instance, soaking and cooking beans can effectively diminish their lectin levels, making them safer for consumption. However, for individuals with sensitivities or health conditions, a diet that minimizes lectin intake may offer considerable relief.

Importance of Dietary Management

Dietary management is critical for maintaining health and preventing chronic diseases. As awareness of food's impact on health continues to grow, more people are exploring dietary strategies that align with their health goals. A low lectin diet can serve as a valuable approach for individuals seeking to manage inflammation, digestive issues, and other health concerns.

Research indicates that dietary changes can lead to significant improvements in symptoms for a variety of conditions. A meta-analysis in the **American Journal of Clinical Nutrition** emphasized the positive effects of diet on chronic inflammation, noting that a diet low in lectins may help reduce inflammatory markers in the body (Johnson et al., 2022).

Implications of Low Lectin Diet on Other Disease Conditions

The implications of a low lectin diet extend to various chronic health conditions, including autoimmune diseases, metabolic syndrome, and cardiovascular issues. Lectins may contribute to the exacerbation of these conditions by promoting inflammation and interfering with nutrient absorption. For example, individuals with autoimmune disorders have reported improved symptoms when adopting a low lectin diet, as highlighted in a review published in **Nutrients**, which noted the potential benefits of reducing dietary lectins (Smith et al., 2020).

By focusing on low lectin foods, individuals can make proactive dietary choices that may help mitigate the impact of these chronic diseases, ultimately leading to improved health outcomes.

How Lectin Intake Affects the Adult Population

In adults, the effects of lectins can vary widely depending on individual sensitivities and overall health. Research shows that some adults may experience heightened sensitivity to lectins, leading to increased gut permeability and inflammation. A study published in the **Journal of

Gastroenterology found that adults with high lectin diets exhibited higher levels of intestinal permeability, which can contribute to a range of health issues, including chronic fatigue and digestive disorders (Baker et al., 2023).

Understanding how lectins affect the adult population is crucial for making informed dietary choices. By adopting a low lectin diet, many individuals have reported improvements in energy levels, digestive health, and overall well-being, highlighting the importance of personalized nutrition in today's health landscape.

As we explore the intricate relationship between diet and health, it becomes evident that understanding the role of lectins is vital for making informed choices. The advancements in research surrounding lectins provide a foundation for why many individuals may benefit from adopting a low lectin diet.

But what exactly are lectins, and how do they impact your health on a deeper level? In the next chapter, we will delve into the fundamentals of lectins—what they are, why they matter, and how they can affect your health. Are you ready to uncover the truth about lectins and their role in your diet? Let's find out in Chapter 3!

Chapter 3: Understanding Lectins

The Impact of a Low Lectin Diet

Recent surveys indicate that approximately **30% of adults** in the United States are actively seeking to modify their diets to reduce inflammation and improve digestive health, with many turning to low lectin diets as a potential solution. As awareness of the effects of dietary lectins grows, more individuals are exploring how eliminating or reducing these proteins can positively impact their overall health.

What Are Lectins?

Lectins are a type of protein found in many plants, particularly in seeds, legumes, and grains. They serve various functions in the plant kingdom, primarily acting as a defense mechanism against pests and diseases. Lectins can bind to carbohydrates, which allows them to interact with cells in the human body. While some lectins are harmless, others can cause adverse effects, particularly when consumed in large quantities or by individuals with specific sensitivities.

Lectins can interfere with nutrient absorption and may contribute to digestive issues. For example, certain types of lectins can bind to the lining of the intestines, potentially leading to increased intestinal permeability— a condition often referred to as "leaky gut." This can result in inflammation and a host of other health issues.

Why Manage Lectin Intake?

Managing lectin intake is important for several reasons:

1.**Digestive Health**: For many individuals, particularly those with existing digestive issues, high lectin foods can exacerbate symptoms such as bloating, gas, and discomfort. Reducing lectin consumption can lead to improved gut health and overall digestive function.

2.**Inflammation Reduction**: Lectins may trigger inflammatory responses in some people, contributing to chronic conditions such as arthritis, autoimmune diseases, and other inflammatory disorders. A low lectin diet may help reduce inflammation and improve symptoms for those affected.

3. **Nutrient Absorption**: Certain lectins can inhibit the absorption of nutrients, leading to deficiencies over time. By managing lectin intake, individuals can enhance their ability to absorb essential vitamins and minerals from food.

4. **Individual Sensitivities**: Some individuals may be more sensitive to lectins than others. For those with specific health concerns, such as irritable bowel syndrome (IBS) or autoimmune conditions, monitoring lectin intake can be a vital part of their dietary management strategy.

Common Sources of Lectins in the Diet

Lectins are found in a wide variety of foods, particularly in:

Legumes: Beans, lentils, and peas are high in lectins, especially when raw or undercooked. Cooking methods, such as soaking and boiling, can significantly reduce their lectin content.

Grains: Whole grains, including wheat, barley, and quinoa, contain lectins. While some grains can be prepared to reduce lectin levels, others may still pose issues for sensitive individuals.

Nightshade Vegetables: Some vegetables, such as tomatoes, potatoes, and eggplants, belong to the nightshade family and contain lectins. These may need to be limited or avoided by those following a low lectin diet.

Dairy Products: Certain dairy products may also contain lectins, particularly those derived from animals fed a grain-based diet.

Nuts and Seeds: While many nuts and seeds are nutritious, some contain lectins that may affect individuals with sensitivities.

By understanding the sources of lectins in the diet, individuals can make informed choices about the foods they consume and take steps to reduce their intake when necessary.

Understanding lectins and their impact on health is crucial for making informed dietary choices. As we continue to explore the effects of lectins on the body, it's important to recognize that not everyone will react the same way to lectins. Individual sensitivities and health conditions play a significant role in how these proteins affect overall well-being.

But how can you effectively navigate your food choices to minimize lectin intake while still enjoying a balanced diet? In the next chapter, we will provide you with a comprehensive low lectin food list, detailing which foods to include and which to avoid. Are you ready to transform your diet with our complete ingredient guide? Let's dive into Chapter 4!

Chapter 4: Low Lectin Food List

Macronutrients and Micronutrients to Consider

When evaluating foods for their lectin content, it's important to consider the following macronutrients and micronutrients:

Protein: Many high-lectin foods, especially legumes and grains, are good sources of plant-based protein. However, other low-lectin protein sources (like grass-fed meats and fish) can provide similar benefits without the negative effects of lectins.

Fiber: While high-lectin foods often contain beneficial fiber, it's essential to balance fiber intake with low-lectin options to ensure digestive health. Low-lectin fruits and vegetables can provide adequate fiber without the associated lectins.

Vitamin C: Fruits and vegetables high in Vitamin C (like bell peppers and citrus fruits) are generally low in lectins and should be included in the diet for their antioxidant properties.

Potassium: Foods rich in potassium (such as leafy greens, cucumbers, and zucchini) are beneficial for maintaining healthy blood pressure and overall health.

Sodium: Be mindful of sodium levels, especially in processed foods. When avoiding high-lectin foods, it's also important to choose low-sodium alternatives to maintain a balanced diet.

Phosphorus: While some high-lectin foods can provide phosphorus, low-lectin alternatives like meats, fish, and dairy can also contribute to your phosphorus intake without the negative effects of lectins.

How to use the charts

The following are my recommended low lectin foods. Refer to the charts to check for the macronutrient and micronutrient values according to the general standard recommendations I have mentioned or as set by your dietitian.

1. The foods are categorized into: Fruits, Vegetables, Grains, Proteins, Dairy & Dairy Alternatives, and Fats & Oils.

2. Each food item is given at least 1 corresponding serving size. We have standardized the serving size to 100 grams, but you will also find other alternative serving sizes to most food items in the charts.

   a. For reference:

G/g = grams	c = cup
mg = milligrams	tsp = teaspoon
svg = serving	tbsp = tablespoon
fl oz = fluid ounce	pc = piece

3. How to read/apply the chart?

   For example, you are only allowed to have around 140mg of Potassium for your snack, and you have 1 peach on hand. Looking at the chart, 1 piece medium-sized raw peach is 150grams, with 285 mg of Potassium. If you have a scale handy, you may want to weigh 75grams only of the peach you have. Or you can just simply slice the peach into half and just eat half of it.

PEACHES	SERVING QUANTITY	SERVING UNIT	CALORIES (kcal)	PROTEIN (g)	TOTAL CARBOHYDRATES (g)	SODIUM (mg)	POTASSIUM (mg)	PHOSPHORUS (mg)	TOTAL FAT (g)
raw, medium	100.00	g	39	0.9	9.5	0.00	190.0	20.00	0.25
approx.	150.00	g	59	1.4	14.3	0.00	285.0	30.00	0.38
	1.00	pc/ item							

4. This chapter ends with a section on High Lectin FOODS TO AVOID. Where I list down foods that you should consume in moderation or better yet complete remove from your diet.

It also goes without saying that though the following chart will give you a general idea of the food that you will be taking in, it's still best to exercise caution and consume them in moderation.

I also would like to emphasize and put heavy stress on consulting with your healthcare team (i.e. your doctor and your nutritionist dietitian) any nutritional and dietary plans that you have, because we are individuals with altogether slightly different needs from one another.

Complete List of Low Lectin Foods

A. FRUITS

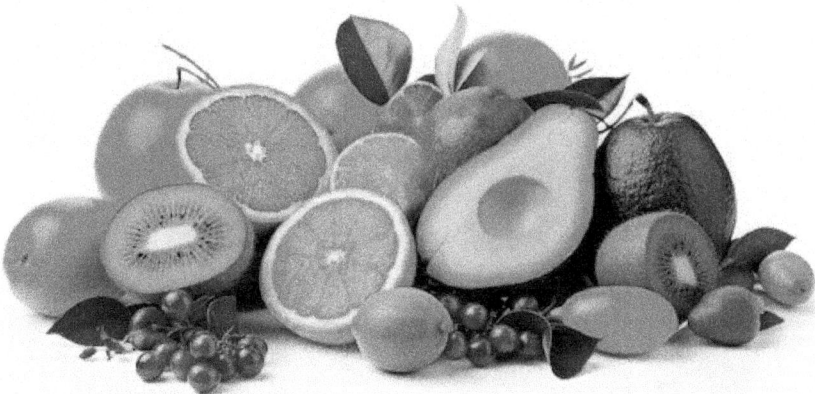

APPLE

	SERVING QUANTITY	SERVING UNIT	CALORIES (kCal)	PROTEIN (g)	TOTAL CARBOHYDRATES (g)	SODIUM (mg)	POTASSIUM (mg)	PHOSPHORUS (mg)	TOTAL FAT (g)
Gala, raw, with skin	100.00	g	57	0.3	13.7	1.00	108.00	11.00	0.12
	172.00	g	98	0.4	23.5	1.72	185.76	18.92	0.21
	1.00	pc, med							
fuji, raw, with skin	100.00	g	63	0.2	15.2	1.00	109.00	13.00	0.18
	192.00	g	121	0.4	29.2	1.92	209.28	24.96	0.35
	1.00	pc, med							
golden delicious, with skin	100.00	g	57	0.3	13.6	2.00	100.00	10.00	0.15
	169.00	g	96	0.5	23.0	3.38	169.00	16.90	0.25
	1.00	pc, med							
granny smith, w/ skin, raw	100.00	g	58	0.4	13.6	1.00	120.00	12.00	0.19
	167.00	g	97	0.7	22.7	1.67	200.40	20.04	0.32
	1.00	pc, med							
juice, frozen concentrate	100.00	g	47	0.1	11.5	7.00	126.00	7.00	0.10
	239.00	g	112	0.3	27.6	16.73	301.14	16.73	0.24
	8.00	fl oz							
applesauce, sweetened, canned	100.00	g	68	0.2	17.5	2.00	75.00	6.00	0.17
	123.00	g	84	0.2	21.5	2.46	92.25	7.38	0.21
	0.50	c							
applesauce, unsweetened, canned	100.00	g	42	0.2	11.3	2.00	74.00	5.00	0.10
	122.00	g	51	0.2	13.8	2.44	90.28	6.10	0.12
	0.50	c							

BLUEBERRIES

	SERVING QUANTITY	SERVING UNIT	CALORIES (kCal)	PROTEIN (g)	TOTAL CARBOHYDRATES (g)	SODIUM (mg)	POTASSIUM (mg)	PHOSPHORUS (mg)	TOTAL FAT (g)
fresh	100.00	g	57	0.7	14.5	1.00	77.00	12.00	0.33
	145.00	g	83	1.1	21.0	1.45	111.6	17.40	0.48
	1.00	c							
sweetened, dried	100.00	g	317	2.5	80.0	3.00	214.0	36.00	2.50
	40.00	g	127	1.0	32.0	1.20	85.60	14.40	1.00
	0.25	c							
wild, frozen	100.00	g	57	0.0	13.9	3.00	68.00	13.00	0.16
	140.00	g	80	0.0	19.4	4.20	95.20	18.20	0.22
	1.00	c							
unsweetened, frozen	100.00	g	51	0.4	12.2	1.00	54.00	11.00	0.64
	155.00	g	79	0.7	18.9	1.55	83.70	17.05	0.99
	1.00	c							
canned, light syrup, drained	100.00	g	88	1.0	22.7	3.00	54.00	12.00	0.40
	244.00	g	215	2.5	55.3	7.32	131.7	29.28	0.98
	1.00	c							

RASP BERRIES / STRAWBERRIES	SERVING QUANTITY	SERVING UNIT	CALORIES (kCal)	PROTEIN (g)	TOTAL CARBOHYDRATES (g)	SODIUM (mg)	POTASSIUM (mg)	PHOSPHORUS (mg)	TOTAL FAT (g)
RASP BERRIES									
raw	100.00	g	52	1.2	11.9	1.00	151.00	29.00	0.69
	123.00	g	64	1.5	14.7	1.23	185.73	35.67	0.80
	1.00	c							
frozen, unsweetend	100.00	g	56	1.2	12.6	4.00	184.00	30.00	0.81
	140.00	g	78	1.6	17.6	5.60	257.60	42.00	1.13
	1.00	c							
red, frozen, sweetened, unthawed	100.00	g	103	0.7	26.2	1.00	114.00	17.00	0.16
	125.00	g	129	0.9	32.7	1.25	142.50	21.25	0.20
	0.50	c							
puree, with seeds	100.00	g	55	na	11.5	4.00	195.00	30.00	0.97
juice concentrate	100.00	g	221	3.0	53.2	10.0	1,178.0	100.0	1.34
STRAWBERRIES									
fresh, whole	100.00	g	32	0.7	7.7	1.00	153.0	24.00	0.30
	144.00	g	46	1.0	11.1	1.44	220.3	34.56	0.43
	1.00	c							
unsweetened, frozen (unthawed)	100.00	g	35	0.4	9.1	2.00	148.0	13.00	0.11
	149.00	g	52	0.6	13.6	2.98	220.5	19.37	
									0.16
	1.00	c							
sweetened, frozen, thawed	100.00	g	78	0.5	21.0	1.00	98.00	12.00	0.14
	127.50	g	99	0.7	26.8	1.28	124.9	15.30	0.18
	0.50	c							
fruit topping	100.00	g	254	0.2	66.3	21.00	51.00	5.00	0.10
	42.00	g	107	0.1	27.9	8.82	21.42	2.10	0.04
	2.00	tbsp							
pastry, 15 pprox, enriched	100.00	g	371	5.4	47.8	445.00	83.00	89.00	18.50
	71.00	g	263	3.8	33.9	315.95	58.93	63.19	13.14
	1.00	pc							
Milkshake (fastfood)	100.00	g	113	3.4	18.9	83.00	182.0	100.0	2.80
	226.40	g	256	7.7	42.8	187.91	412.1	226.4	6.34
	8.00	fl oz							
yogurt 15ppro, low fat	100.00	g	105	8.2	12.3	33.00	129.0	109.0	2.57
1 item = 1 container	150.00	g	158	12.3	18.4	49.50	193.5	163.5	3.86
	1.00	item							

CHERRIES	SERVING QUANTITY	SERVING UNIT	CALORIES (kcal)	PROTEIN (g)	TOTAL CARBOHYDRATES (g)	SODIUM (mg)	POTASSIUM (mg)	PHOSPHORUS (mg)	TOTAL FAT (g)
sweet, without	100.00	g	63	1.1	16.0	0.00	222.0	21.00	0.20
pits	154.00	g	97	1.6	24.7	0.00	341.9	32.34	0.31
	1.00	c							
sour red, without	100.00	g	50	1.0	12.2	3.00	173.0	15.00	0.30
pits	155.00	g	78	1.6	18.9	4.65	268.2	23.25	0.47
	1.00	c							
juice, tart	100.00	g	59	0.3	13.7	4.00	161.0	17.00	0.54
	269.00	g	159	0.8	36.9	10.76	433.1	45.73	1.45
	1.00	c							
Pitanga or	100.00	g	33	0.8	7.5	3.00	103.0	11.00	0.40
Surinam	173.00	g	57	1.4	13.0	5.19	178.2	19.03	0.69
	1.00	c							
tart, dried,	100.00	g	333	1.3	80.5	13.00	376.0	36.00	0.73
sweetened	40.00	g	133	0.5	32.2	5.20	150.4	14.40	0.29
	0.25	c							
maraschino,	100.00	g	165	0.2	42.0	4.00	21.0	3.00	0.21
canned, drained	5.00	g	8	0.0	2.1	0.20	1.05	0.15	0.01
	1.00	pc/ item							
sweet, canned in	100.00	g	54	0.9	13.8	3.00	131.0	22.00	0.02
juice, pitted	250.00	g	135	2.3	34.5	7.50	327.5	55.00	0.05
	1.00	c							
sweet, canned in	100.00	g	46	0.8	11.8	1.00	131.0	15.00	0.13
water	248.00	g	114	1.9	29.2	2.48	324.9	37.20	0.32
	1.00	c							
sweet, frozen,	100.00	g	89	1.2	22.4	1.00	199.0	16.00	0.13
sweetened	259.00	g	231	3.0	57.9	2.59	515.4	41.44	0.34
thawed	1.00	c							
pie filling, canned	100.00	g	115	0.4	28.0	18.00	105.0	15.00	0.07
1/8 of 21 oz can	74.00	g	85	0.3	20.7	13.32	77.70	11.10	0.05
	1.00	svg							
pie fillings, low	100.00	g	53	0.8	12.0	12.00	118.0	15.00	0.16
calorie	264.00	g	140	2.2	31.6	31.68	311.5	39.60	0.42
	1.00	c							
sour red, canned	100.00	g	42	0.7	10.5	4.00	115.0	16.00	0.21
in water, drained	168.00	g	71	1.2	17.6	6.72	193.2	26.88	0.35
	1.00	c							
sour red,	100.00	g	46	0.9	11.0	1.00	124.0	16.00	0.44
16pprox.16ned,	155.00	g	71	1.4	17.1	1.55	192.2	24.80	0.68
frozen									
unthawed	1.00	c							
sour red, canned	100.00	g	75	0.7	19.3	7.00	95.00	10.00	0.10
in light syrup	126.00	g	95	0.9	24.3	8.82	119.7	12.60	0.13
	0.50	c							

CANTALOUPE MELON	SERVING QUANTITY	SERVING UNIT	CALORIES (kCal)	PROTEIN (g)	TOTAL CARBOHYDRATES (g)	SODIUM (mg)	POTASSIUM (mg)	PHOSPHORUS (mg)	TOTAL FAT (g)
composite, raw	100.00	g	31	0.7	7.5	8.22	202.4	8.67	0.20
	165.50	g	51	1.1	12.5	13.60	334.9	14.34	0.33
	1.00	c							
honeydew, balls	100.00	g	36	0.5	9.1	18.00	228.0	11.00	0.14
1 slice = 125g	132.75	g	48	0.7	12.1	23.90	302.7	14.60	0.19
	0.75	c							
Navajo	100.00	g	21	0.8	4.1	11.00	140.0	9.00	0.20
	85.05	g	18	0.7	3.5	9.36	119.1	7.65	0.17
	3.00	oz							
melon balls, frozen, unthawed	100.00	g	33	0.8	7.9	31.00	280.0	12.00	0.25
	173.00	g	57	1.5	13.7	53.63	484.4	20.76	0.43
	1.00	c							

GRAPE-FRUIT

	SERVING QUANTITY	SERVING UNIT	CALORIES (kCal)	PROTEIN (g)	TOTAL CARBOHYDRATES (g)	SODIUM (mg)	POTASSIUM (mg)	PHOSPHORUS (mg)	TOTAL FAT (g)
fresh	100.00	g	32	0.6	8.1	0.00	139.0	8.00	0.10
	153.33	g	49	1.0	12.4	0.00	213.1	12.27	0.15
	0.67	c							
white, fresh, small (3.5 diameter)	100.00	g	33	0.7	8.4	0.00	148.0	8.00	0.10
	118.00	g	39	0.8	9.9	0.00	174.6	9.44	0.12
	0.50	pc							
pink or red	100.00	g	42	0.8	10.7	0.00	135.0	18.00	0.14
	153.33	g	64	1.2	16.4	0.00	207.0	27.60	0.21
	0.67	c							
juice, white	100.00	g	39	0.5	9.2	1.00	162.0	15.00	0.10
	247.00	g	96	1.2	22.7	2.47	400.2	37.05	0.25
	8.00	fl oz							
juice, pink	100.00	g	39	0.5	9.2	1.00	162.0	15.00	0.10
	247.00	g	96	1.2	22.7	2.47	400.2	37.05	0.25
	1.00	c							
juice, unsweetened, pink, canned	100.00	g	37	0.6	7.5	2.00	141.0	17.00	0.66
	247.20	g	91	1.4	18.6	4.94	348.6	42.02	1.63
	8.00	fl oz							

GRAPE

GRAPE	SERVING QUANTITY	SERVING UNIT	CALORIES (kCal)	PROTEIN (g)	TOTAL CARBOHYDRATES (g)	SODIUM (mg)	POTASSIUM (mg)	PHOSPHORUS (mg)	TOTAL FAT (g)
red or green, seedless	100.00	g	69	0.7	18.1	2.00	191.00	20.00	0.16
	151.00	g	104	1.1	27.3	3.02	288.41	30.20	0.24
	1.00	c							
juice, unsweetened, plus Vit.C	100.00	g	60	0.4	14.8	5.00	104.00	14.00	0.13
	252.80	g	152	0.9	37.3	12.64	262.90	35.39	0.33
	8.00	fl oz							
fruit mixed/ fruit cocktail, light, drained	100.00	g	55	0.4	14.3	6.00	85.00	13.00	0.08
juice, sweetened, frozen concentrate 6 fl oz can	100.00	g	179	0.7	44.4	7.00	74.00	15.00	0.31
	216.00	g	387	1.4	95.8	15.12	159.84	32.40	0.67
	1.00	can/ item							
seedless, Thompson, canned in water	100.00	g	40	0.5	10.3	6.00	107.00	18.00	0.11
	245.00	g	98	1.2	25.2	14.70	262.15	44.10	0.27
	1.00	c							
jelly 1 packet= 14g (0.5oz)	100.00	g	266	0.2	70.0	30.00	54.00	6.00	0.02
	21.00	g	56	0.0	14.7	6.30	11.34	1.26	0.00
	1	tbsp							
KIWI (Chinese gooseberries)									
fresh, medium, without skin	100.00	g	61	1.1	14.7	3.00	312.0	34.00	0.52
	76.00	g	46	0.9	11.1	2.28	237.1	25.84	0.40
	1.00	pc							

LEMON	SERVING QUANTITY	SERVING UNIT	CALORIES (kcal)	PROTEIN (g)	TOTAL CARBOHYDRATES (g)	SODIUM (mg)	POTASSIUM (mg)	PHOSPHORUS (mg)	TOTAL FAT (g)
whole, without seeds	100	g	20	1.2	10.7	3.00	145.0	15.00	0.30
	108.00	g	22	1.3	11.6	3.24	156.6	16.20	0.32
	1.00	pc/ item							
peeled, 2-1/8" in diameter)	100.00	g	29	1.1	9.3	2.00	138.0	16.00	0.30
	58.00	g	17	0.6	5.4	1.16	80.04	9.28	0.17
	1.00	pc/ item							
juice, fresh	100.00	g	22	0.4	6.9	1.00	103.0	8.00	0.24
	30.50	g	7	0.1	2.1	0.31	31.42	2.44	0.07
	1.00	fl oz							
peel or zest	100.00	g	47	1.5	16.0	6.00	160.0	12.00	0.30
	2.00	g	1	0.0	0.3	0.12	3.20	0.24	0.01
	1.00	tsp							
pudding mix	100.00	g	363	0.1	91.8	506.00	5.00	3.00	0.50
1 svg = ½ c 1 package = 85g	21.20	g	77	0.0	19.5	107.27	1.06	0.64	0.11
	1.00	svg							
juice, canned	100.00	g	17	0.5	5.6	24.00	109.0	9.00	0.07
	30.50	g	5	0.1	1.7	7.32	33.25	2.75	0.02
	1.00	fl oz							
soda, lemon lime	100.00	g	40	0.1	24.9	9.00	1.00	0.00	0.02
	245.60	g	98	0.1	10.1	22.10	2.46	0.00	0.05
	8.00	fl oz							
juice, unsweetened, frozen	100.00	g	22	0.5	6.5	1.00	89.00	8.00	0.32
	5.08	g	1	0.0	0.3	0.05	4.52	0.41	0.02
	1.00	tsp							
pudding, ready to eat	100.00	g	125	0.1	25.0	140.00	1.00	5.00	3.00
1 can= 5 oz	142.00	g	178	0.1	35.5	198.80	1.42	7.10	4.26
	1.00	can/ item							
tea, black, sweetened, ready to drink	100.00	g	45	0.0	10.8	3.00	14.00	1.00	0.22
	271.00	g	122	0.0	29.3	8.13	37.94	2.71	0.60
	1.00	c							

ORANGE

	SERVING QUANTITY	SERVING UNIT	CALORIES (kcal)	PROTEIN (g)	TOTAL CARBOHYDRATES (g)	SODIUM (mg)	POTASSIUM (mg)	PHOSPHORUS (mg)	TOTAL FAT (g)
whole, 2-5/8"	100.00	g	47	0.9	11.8	0.00	181.0	14.00	0.12
diameter	131.00	g	62	1.2	15.4	0.00	237.1	18.34	0.16
	1.00	pc/ item							
Valencia	100.00	g	49	1.0	11.9	0.00	179.0	17.00	0.30
(California)	135.00	g	66	1.4	16.1	0.00	241.7	22.95	0.41
	0.75	c							
Navel (California)	100.00	g	49	0.9	12.5	1.00	166.0	28.46	0.15
	123.75	g	61	1.1	15.5	1.24	205.4	23.00	0.19
	0.75	c							
Clementines	100.00	g	47	0.9	12.0	1.00	177.0	21.00	0.15
	74.00	g	35	0.6	8.9	0.74	130.9	15.54	0.11
	1.00	pc/ item							
orange sections	100.00	g	47	0.9	11.8	0.00	181.0	14.00	0.12
	135.00	g	63	1.3	15.9	0.00	244.4	18.90	0.16
	0.75	c							
juice	100.00	g	45	0.7	10.4	1.00	200.0	17.00	0.20
	248.00	g	112	1.7	25.8	2.48	496.0	42.16	0.50
	8.00	fl oz							
Florida, sections	100.00	g	46	0.7	11.5	0.00	169.0	12.00	0.21
1 fruit = 141g	138.75	g	64	1.0	16.0	0.00	234.5	16.65	0.29
	0.75	c							
soda	100.00	g	48	0.0	12.3	12.00	2.00	1.00	0.00
	248.00	g	119	0.0	30.5	29.76	4.96	2.48	0.00
	8.00	fl oz							
marmalade	100.00	g	246	0.3	66.3	56.00	37.00	4.00	0.00
	20.00	g	49	0.1	13.3	11.20	7.40	0.80	0.00
	1.00	tbsp							
juice, frozen	100.00	g	95	0.5	23.2	8.00	100.0	13.00	0.00
	238.40	g	70	0.4	17.2	5.92	74.00	9.62	0.00
	1.00	c							
orange peel zest	100.00	g	97	1.5	25.0	3.00	212.0	21.00	0.20
	2.00	g	2	0.0	0.5	0.06	4.24	0.42	0.00
	1.00	tsp							
juice,	100.00	g	47	0.7	11.0	4.00	184.0	17.00	0.15
unsweetened,	249.00	g	117	1.7	27.4	9.96	458.2	42.33	0.37
canned	8.00	fl oz							
Mandarin, canned	100.00	g		37	0.6	9.6	5.00	133.0	10.00
in juice	249.00	g		92	1.5	23.8	12.45	331.2	24.90
	1.00	c							
juice, light, no	100.00	g		21	0.2	5.4	4.00	188.0	4.00
pulp	240.00	g		50	0.5	13.0	9.60	451.2	9.60
	8.00	fl oz							
Mandarin, canned	100.00	g		61	0.5	16.2	6.00	78.00	10.00
in light syrup	252.00	g		154	1.1	40.8	15.12	196.6	25.20
	1.00	c							

20

PEACHES

PEACHES	SERVING QUANTITY	SERVING UNIT	CALORIES (kcal)	PROTEIN (g)	TOTAL CARBOHYDRATES (g)	SODIUM (mg)	POTASSIUM (mg)	PHOSPHORUS (mg)	TOTAL FAT (g)
raw, medium	100.00	g	39	0.9	9.5	0.00	190.0	20.00	0.25
(21pprox. 4/lb)	150.00	g	59	1.4	14.3	0.00	285.0	30.00	0.38
	1.00	pc/ item							
dried	100.00	g	325	4.9	83.2	10.00	1,351	162.0	1.03
	38.67	g	126	1.9	32.2	3.87	522.4	62.64	0.40
	0.33	c							
slices	100.00	g	39	0.9	9.5	0.00	190.0	20.00	0.25
	154.00	g	60	1.4	14.7	0.00	292.6	30.80	0.39
	1.00	c							
nectar, canned	100.00	g	49	0.1	11.6	11.00	30.00	3.00	0.57
	249.00	g	122	0.3	28.9	27.39	74.70	7.47	1.42
	8.00	fl oz							
pie, prepared	100.00	g	224	1.9	33.0	217.00	125.0	22.00	10.00
1/6 of 8-in. pie	117.00	g	262	2.2	38.5	253.89	146.3	25.74	11.70
	1.00	slice							
slices, sweetened, frozen	100.00	g	94	0.6	24.0	6.00	130.0	11.00	0.13
	125.00	g	118	0.8	30.0	7.50	162.5	13.75	0.16
	0.50	c							
halves/ slices, canned in water	100.00	g	24	0.4	6.1	3.00	99.00	10.00	0.06
	122.00	g	29	0.5	7.5	3.66	120.8	12.20	0.07
	0.50	c							
halves/ slices, canned in juice	100.00	g	44	0.6	11.6	4.00	128.0	17.00	0.03
	124.00	g	55	0.8	14.4	4.96	158.7	21.08	0.04
	0.50	c							
canned in extra light syrup	100.00	g	42	0.4	11.1	5.00	74.00	11.00	0.10
	123.50	g	52	0.5	13.7	6.18	91.39	13.59	0.12
	0.50	c							
canned in heavy syrup	100.00	g	75	0.4	20.1	4.00	85.00	9.00	0.10
	242.00	g	182	1.0	48.6	9.68	205.7	21.78	0.24
	1.00	c							
canned in light syrup, drained	100.00	g	61	0.6	15.7	7.00	87.00	10.00	0.15
fruit cocktail, canned light syrup with solids and liquid	100.00	g	55	0.4	14.3	6.00	85.00	13.00	0.08

LIME	SERVING QUANTITY	SERVING UNIT	CALORIES (kcal)	PROTEIN (g)	TOTAL CARBOHYDRATES (g)	SODIUM (mg)	POTASSIUM (mg)	PHOSPHORUS (mg)	TOTAL FAT (g)
whole, 2" in diameter	100.00	g	30	0.7	10.5	2.00	102.0	18.00	0.20
	67.00	g	20	0.5	7.1	1.34	68.34	12.06	0.13
	1.00	pc/ item							
juice, fresh	100.00	g	25	0.4	8.4	2.00	117.0	14.00	0.07
	5.13	g	1	0.0	0.4	0.10	6.01	0.72	0.00
	1.00	tsp							
juice, unsweetened, canned	100.00	g	21	0.3	6.7	16.00	75.00	10.00	0.23
	246.00	g	52	0.6	16.5	39.36	184.5	24.60	0.57
	1.00	c							
frozen ice dessert	100.00	g	128	0.4	32.6	22.00	3.00	1.00	0.00
	99.00	g	127	0.4	32.3	21.78	2.97	0.99	0.00
	0.50	c							
PEARS									
whole, medium (2.5/lb)	100.00	g	57	0.4	15.2	1.00	116.00	16.00	0.14
	166.00	g	95	0.6	25.3	1.66	192.56	19.92	0.23
	1.00	pc							
halves, canned in water	100.00	g	29	0.2	7.8	2.00	53.00	7.00	0.03
	244.00	g	71	0.5	19.1	4.88	129.32	17.08	0.07
	1.00	c							
Asian	100.00	g	42	0.5	10.7	0.00	121.00	11.00	0.23
	122.00	g	51	0.6	13.0	0.00	147.62	13.42	0.28
	1.00	pc							

PINE APPLE

	SERVING QUANTITY	SERVING UNIT	CALORIES (kCal)	PROTEIN (g)	TOTAL CARBOHYDRATES (g)	SODIUM (mg)	POTASSIUM (mg)	PHOSPHORUS (mg)	TOTAL FAT (g)
traditional varieties, diced	100.00	g	45	0.6	18.3	1.00	125.00	9.00	0.13
	155.00	g	70	0.9	11.8	1.55	193.75	13.95	0.20
	1.00	c							
sweetened, frozen, chunks	100.00	g	86	0.4	22.2	2.00	100.00	4.00	0.10
	245.00	g	211	1.0	54.4	4.90	245.00	9.80	0.25
	1.00	c							
canned in water crushed, sliced or chunks	100.00	g	32	0.4	8.3	1.00	127.00	4.00	0.09
	246.00	g	79	1.1	20.4	2.46	312.42	9.84	0.22
	1.00	c							
canned in juice crushed, sliced, or chunks	100.00	g	60	0.4	15.7	1.00	122.00	6.00	0.08
	249.00	g	149	1.1	39.1	2.49	303.78	14.94	0.20
	1.00	c							
extra sweet variety, diced	100.00	g	51	0.5	13.5	1.00	108.00	8.00	0.11
	155.00	g	79	0.8	20.9	1.55	167.40	12.40	0.17
	1.00	c							
juice, unsweetened, canned	100.00	g	53	0.4	12.9	2.00	130.00	8.00	0.12
	250.00	g	133	0.9	32.2	5.00	325.00	20.00	0.30
	8.00	fl oz							
canned in light syrup crushed, sliced, or chunks	100.00	g	52	0.4	13.5	1.00	105.00	7.00	0.12
	126.00	g	66	0.5	17.0	1.26	132.30	8.82	0.15
	0.50	c							
juice, unsweetened, frozen concentrate	100.00	g	179	1.3	44.3	3.00	472.00	28.00	0.10
	288.00	g	387	2.8	95.7	6.48	1,019.5	60.48	0.22
	1.00	c							
juice, 23pprox.23ned with Vit A, C & E	100.00	g	50	0.4	12.2	3.00	132.00	9.00	0.14
	250.00	g	125	0.9	30.5	7.50	330.00	22.50	0.35
	1.00	c							

PLUM

	SERVING QUANTITY	SERVING UNIT	CALORIES (kCal)	PROTEIN (g)	TOTAL CARBOHYDRATES (g)	SODIUM (mg)	POTASSIUM (mg)	PHOSPHORUS (mg)	TOTAL FAT (g)
whole, fresh, sliced	100.00	g	46	0.7	11.4	0.00	157.0	16.00	0.28
	165.00	g	76	1.2	18.8	0.00	259.1	26.40	0.46
	1.00	c							
sauce	100.00	g	184	0.9	42.8	538.00	259.0	22.00	1.04
	19.00	g	35	0.2	8.1	102.22	49.21	4.18	0.20
	1.00	tbsp							
purple, pitted, canned in water	100.00	g	41	0.4	11.0	1.00	126.0	13.00	0.01
	249.00	g	102	1.0	27.5	2.49	313.7	32.37	0.02
	1.00	c							
purple, canned in juice	100.00	g	58	0.5	15.2	1.00	154.0	15.00	0.02
	252.00	g	146	1.3	38.2	2.52	388.1	37.80	0.05
	1.00	c							

WATER MELON	SERVING QUANTITY	SERVING UNIT	CALORIES (kCal)	PROTEIN (g)	TOTAL CARBOHYDRATES (g)	SODIUM (mg)	POTASSIUM (mg)	PHOSPHORUS (mg)	TOTAL FAT (g)
raw, balls	100.00	g	30	0.6	7.6	1.00	112.00	11.00	0.15
	154.00	g	46	0.9	11.6	1.54	172.00	16.00	0.23
	1.00	c							
juice, 100%, no	100.00	g	30	0.6	7.6	1.00	112.00	11.00	0.15
ice	30.00	g	9	0.2	2.3	0.30	33.60	3.30	0.05
	1.00	fl oz							
seeds, kernels,	100.00	g	557	28.3	15.3	99.00	648.00	755.0	47.37
dried	28.35	g	158	8.0	4.3	28.10	184.00	214.0	13.40
	1.00	oz							

B. VEGETABLES

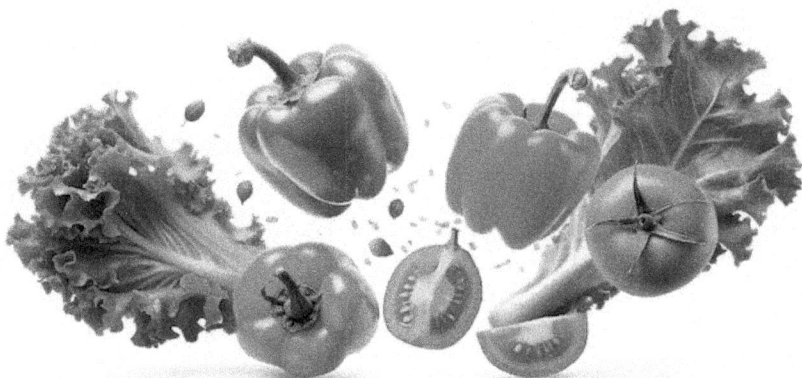

	SERVING QUANTITY	SERVING UNIT	CALORIES (kCal)	PROTEIN (g)	TOTAL CARBOHYDRATES (g)	SODIUM (mg)	POTASSIUM (mg)	PHOSPHORUS (mg)	TOTAL FAT (g)
ARUGULA									
raw, leaves	100	g	25	2.6	3.7	27.00	369	52.00	0.66
	80.00	g	20	2.1	2.9	21.60	295	41.60	0.53
	4.00	c							
salad mixed	100	g	18	1.5	3.3	16.94	299	32.15	0.27
baby greens	41.25	g	7	0.6	1.4	6.99	123	13.26	0.11
Arugula,butterhead, endives, Radicchio	1.00	c							
ASPARAGUS									
boiled, drained	100.00	g	22	2.4	4.1	14.00	224.00	54.00	0.22
	90.00	g	20	2.2	3.7	12.60	201.60	48.60	0.20
	0.50	c							
frozen	100.00	g	24	3.2	4.1	8.00	253.00	64.00	0.23
	87.00	g	21	2.8	3.6	6.96	220.11	55.68	0.20
	6.00	pcs							
frozen, boiled,	100.00	g	18	3.0	1.9	3.00	172.00	49.00	0.42
drained	90.00	g	16	2.7	1.7	2.70	154.80	44.10	0.38
	0.50	c							
canned,	100.00	g	19	2.1	2.5	287.00	172.00	43.00	0.65
drained	121.00	g	23	2.6	3.0	347.27	208.12	52.03	0.79
	0.50	c							
BROCCOLI									
florets, raw	100.00	g	28	3.0	5.1	27.00	325.00	66.00	0.35
	71.00	g	20	2.1	3.6	19.17	230.75	46.86	0.25
	1.00	c							
Cooked, no salt	100.00	g	35	2.4	7.2	41.00	293.00	67.00	0.41
	78.00	g	27	1.9	5.6	31.98	228.54	52.26	0.32
	0.50	c							
frozen, spears	100.00	g	29	3.1	5.4	17.00	250.00	59.00	0.34
	85.05	g	25	2.6	4.6	14.46	212.62	50.18	0.29
	3.00	oz							
BRUSSEL SPROUTS									
raw	100.00	g	43	33.4	9.0	25.00	389.00	69.00	0.30
	88.00	g	38	3.0	7.9	22.00	342.00	60.70	0.26
	1.00	c							

PEPPER

	SERVING QUANTITY	SERVING UNIT	CALORIES (kCal)	PROTEIN (g)	TOTAL CARBOHYDRATES (g)	SODIUM (mg)	POTASSIUM (mg)	PHOSPHORUS (mg)	TOTAL FAT (g)
bell, sweet	100.00	g	27	1.0	6.3	2.00	212.00	24.00	
yellow, 3 in	186.00	g	50	1.9	11.8	3.72	394.32	44.64	
diameter	1.00	pc							
bell, sweet	100.00	g	20	0.9	4.6	3.00	175.00	20.00	
green, chopped	74.50	g	15	0.6	3.5	2.24	130.38	14.90	
	0.50	c							
bell, sweet green, sauteed	100.00	g	116	0.8	4.2	17.00	134.00	15.00	
bell, sweet red,	100.00	g	26	1.0	6.0	4.00	211.00	26.00	
chopped	74.50	g	19	0.7	4.5	2.98	157.20	19.37	
	0.50	c							
bell, sweet red, sauteed	100.00	g	133	1.0	6.6	21.00	193.00	23.00	
bell, sweet red,	100.00	g	16	1.0	3.3	4.00	72.00	13.00	
chopped, frozen,	85.05	g	14	0.8	2.8	3.40	61.24	11.06	
drained, boiled, no salt added	3.00	oz							
jalapeno, sliced	100.00	g	29	0.9	6.5	3.00	248.00	26.00	
	22.50	g	7	0.2	1.5	0.68	55.80	5.85	
	0.13	c							
serrano,	100.00	g	32	1.7	6.7	10.00	305.00	40.00	
chopped	26.25	g	8	0.5	1.8	2.63	80.06	10.50	
	0.25	c							
black, ground	100.00	g	251	10.4	64.0	20.00	1,329.00	158.00	
	2.10	g	5	0.2	1.3	0.42	27.91	3.32	
	1.00	tsp							
white, ground	100.00	g	296	10.4	68.6	5.00	73.00	176.00	
	2.40	g	7	0.3	1.7	0.12	1.75	4.22	
	1.00	tsp							
hot chilli, red	100.00	g	40	1.9	8.8	9.00	322.00	43.00	
	45.00	g	18	0.8	4.0	4.05	144.90	19.35	
	1.00	pc							

ZUCCHINI

	SERVING QUANTITY	SERVING UNIT	CALORIES (kCal)	PROTEIN (g)	TOTAL CARBOHYDRATES (g)	SODIUM (mg)	POTASSIUM (mg)	PHOSPHORUS (mg)	TOTAL FAT (g)
Raw include skin	100	g	17	1.21	3.11	8.0	261.0	38	0.32
sliced	113	g	19.2	1.37	3.51	9.04	295	42.9	0.362
	1	c							

CARROTS

	SERVING QUANTITY	SERVING UNIT	CALORIES (kcal)	PROTEIN (g)	TOTAL CARBOHYDRATES (g)	SODIUM (mg)	POTASSIUM (mg)	PHOSPHORUS (mg)	TOTAL FAT (g)
strips, slices	100.0	g	41	0.9	9.6	69.00	320.0	35.00	
	122.0	g	50	1.1	11.7	84.18	390.4	42.70	
	1.00	c							
grated	100.0	g	41	0.9	9.6	69.00	320.0	35.00	
	82.50	g	34	0.8	7.9	56.93	264.0	28.88	
	0.75	c							
sliced,boileddrained, no salt	100.0	g	35	0.8	8.2	58.00	235.0	30.00	
	78.00	g	27	0.6	6.4	45.24	183.3	23.40	
	0.50	c							
frozen	100.0	g	36	0.8	7.9	68.00	235.0	33.00	
	85.33	g	31	0.7	6.7	58.03	200.5	28.16	
	0.67	c							
baby	100.0	g	35	0.6	8.2	78.00	237.0	28.00	
	80.00	g	28	0.5	6.6	62.40	189.6	22.40	
	8.00	pcs							
juice, canned	100.0	g	40	1.0	9.3	66.00	292.0	42.00	
	236.00	g	94	2.2	21.9	155.76	689.1	99.12	
	8.00	fl oz							

CAULIFLOWER

green,raw	100.0	g	31	3.0	6.1	23.00	300.0	62.00	0.30
	64.00	g	20	1.9	3.9	14.72	192.0	39.68	0.19
	1.00	c							
cooked, no salt	100.0	g	32	3.0	6.3	23.00	278.0	57.00	0.31
	62.00	g	20	1.9	3.9	14.26	172.3	35.34	0.19
	0.50	c							

CUCUMBER

sliced, raw	100.0	g	15	0.7	3.6	2.00	147.0	24.00	0.11
	52.00	g	8	0.3	1.9	1.04	76.44	12.48	0.06
	0.50	c							
sliced	100.0	g	15	0.7	3.6	2.00	147.0	24.00	0.11
	78.00	g	12	0.5	2.8	1.56	114.6	18.72	0.09
	0.75	c							

EGGPLANT AUBERGINE	SERVING QUANTITY	SERVING UNIT	CALORIES (kCal)	PROTEIN (g)	TOTAL CARBOHYDRATES (g)	SODIUM (mg)	POTASSIUM (mg)	PHOSPHORUS (mg)	TOTAL FAT (g)
boiled, drained,	100.0	g	35	0.8	8.7	1.00	123.0	15.00	0.23
no salt	99.00	g	35	0.8	8.6	0.99	121.7	14.85	0.23
cut in 1" cubes	1.00	c							
pickled	100.0	g	49	0.9	9.8	1,674	12.00	9.00	0.70
	136	g	67	1.2	13.3	2,276	16.32	12.24	0.95
	1.00	c							
BEANS									
green wax, raw	100.0	g	31	1.8	7.0	6.00	211.0	38.00	
	82.50	g	26	1.5	5.8	4.95	174.1	31.35	
	0.75	c							
green wax,	100.0	g	33	1.8	7.5	3.00	186.0	32.00	
frozen	82.67	g	27	1.5	6.2	2.48	153.7	26.45	
	0.67	c							
green wax, boiled,	100.0	g	35	1.9	7.9	1.00	146.0	29.00	
drained	125.0	g	44	2.4	9.9	1.25	182.5	36.25	
	1.00	c							
green wax, canned,	100.0	g	21	1.1	4.2	268.00	96.00	22.00	
drained	135.0	g	28	1.4	5.7	361.80	129.6	29.70	
	1.00	c							
KALE									
raw, chopped	100.0	g	35	2.9	4.4	53.00	348.0	55.00	1.49
	83.75	g	29	2.5	3.7	44.39	291.4	46.06	1.25
	1.25	c							
chopped, boiled,	100.0	g	36	2.9	5.3	16.00	144.0	42.00	1.21
drained, no salt	65.00	g	23	1.9	3.5	10.40	93.6	27.30	0.79
	0.50	c							
scotch, raw,	100.0	g	42	2.8	8.3	70.00	450.0	62.00	0.60
chopped	83.75	g	35	2.4	7.0	58.63	376.8	51.93	0.50
	1.25	c							
scotch, boiled,	100.0	g	28	1.9	5.6	45.00	274.0	38.00	0.41
drained, chopped no salt	86.67	g	24	1.7	4.9	39.00	237.4	32.93	0.36
	0.67	c							
frozen, raw	100.0	g	28	2.7	4.9	15.00	333.0	29.00	0.46
1 pack=10 oz/ 284g	85.05	g	24	2.3	4.2	12.76	283.2	24.66	0.39
	3.00	oz							
frozen, chopped,	100.0	g	36	2.9	5.3	16.00	144.0	42.00	1.21
boiled, drained,	65.00	g	23	1.9	3.5	10.40	93.60	27.30	0.79
no salt	0.50	c							

LETTUCE

	SERVING QUANTITY	SERVING UNIT	CALORIES (kcal)	PROTEIN (g)	TOTAL CARBOHYDRATES (g)	SODIUM (mg)	POTASSIUM (mg)	PHOSPHORUS (mg)	TOTAL FAT (g)
romaine,	100.0	g	17	1.2	3.3		8.00	247.0	30.00
shredded	70.50	g	12	0.9	2.3		5.64	174.1	21.15
	1.50	c							
butterhead,	100.0	g	13	1.4	2.2		5.00	238.0	33.00
medium leaves	82.50	g	11	1.1	1.8		4.13	196.3	27.23
	11.00	pcs							
Red Leaf,	100.0	g	13	1.3	2.3		25	187	28.00
shredded	28.00	g	4	0.4	0.6		7	52.36	7.84
	1.00	c							
Iceberg, shredded	100.0	g	14	0.9	3.0		10	141	20.00
or chopped	108.0	g	15	1.0	3.2		11	152.2	21.60
	1.50	c							
Iceberg, loose	100.0	g	14	0.9	3.0		10	141.0	20.00
leaves, medium	80.00	g	11	0.7	2.4		8	112.8	16.00
	10.00	pcs							

RADISH

	SERVING QUANTITY	SERVING UNIT	CALORIES (kcal)	PROTEIN (g)	TOTAL CARBOHYDRATES (g)	SODIUM (mg)	POTASSIUM (mg)	PHOSPHORUS (mg)	TOTAL FAT (g)
oriental (Daikon),	100.0	g	18	0.6	4.1	21.00	227.0	23.00	0.10
7" long	338.0	g	61	2.0	13.9	70.98	767.2	77.74	0.34
	1.00	pc							
oriental, boiled,	100.0	g	17	0.7	3.4	13.00	285.0	24.00	0.24
drained, no salt									
sliced	73.50	g	13	0.5	2.5	9.56	209.4	17.64	0.18
	0.50	c							
sprouts	100.0	g	43	3.8	3.6	6.00	86.00	113.0	2.53
	38.00	g	16	1.5	1.4	2.28	32.68	42.94	0.96
	1.00	c							

SPINACH

	SERVING QUANTITY	SERVING UNIT	CALORIES (kcal)	PROTEIN (g)	TOTAL CARBOHYDRATES (g)	SODIUM (mg)	POTASSIUM (mg)	PHOSPHORUS (mg)	TOTAL FAT (g)
raw, chopped	100.0	g	23	2.9	3.6	79.00	558.0	49.00	0.39
	90.00	g	21	2.6	3.3	71.10	502.2	44.10	0.35
	3.00	c							
frozen	100.0	g	29	3.6	4.2	74.00	346.0	49.00	0.57
	78.00	g	23	2.8	3.3	57.72	269.8	38.22	0.44
	0.50	c							
chopped, boiled,	100.0	g	23	3.0	3.8	70.00	466.0	56.00	0.26
drained, no salt	90.00	g	21	2.7	3.4	63.00	419.4	50.40	0.23
	0.50	c							
mustard	100.0	g	22	2.2	3.9	21.00	449.0	28.00	0.30
(Tendergreens)	150.0	g	33	3.3	5.9	31.50	673.5	42.00	0.45
	1.00	c							
mustard, boiled,	100.0	g	16	1.7	2.8	14.00	285.0	18.00	0.20
drained, no salt	180.0	g	29	3.1	5.0	25.20	513.0	32.40	0.36
	1.00	c							

C. GRAINS

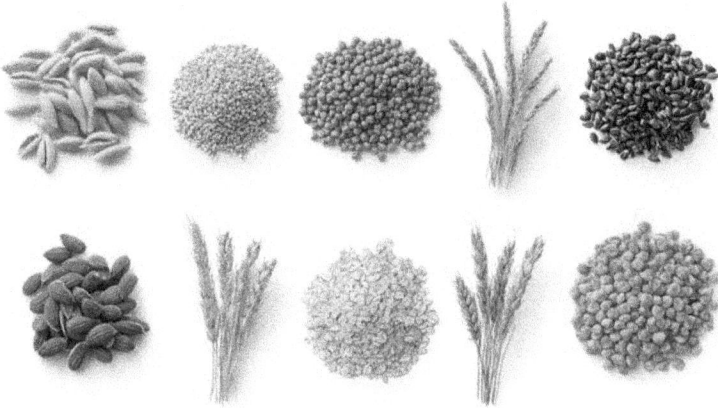

31

RICE	SERVING QUANTITY	SERVING UNIT	CALORIES (kcal)	PROTEIN (g)	TOTAL CARBOHYDRATES (g)	SODIUM (mg)	POTASSIUM (mg)	PHOSPHORUS (mg)	TOTAL FAT (g)
white, unenriched	100.0	g	359	6.9	79.8	5.00	75.00	94.00	1.30
white, cooked, glutinous	100.0	g	96	2.0	21.0	5.00	20.00	33.00	0.27
	174.0	g	167	3.5	36.5	6.60	26.40	43.60	0.36
	1.00	c							
white, long-grain, parboiled enriched, cooked	100.0	g	123	2.9	26.1	0.00	29.00	37.00	0.21
	158.0	g	194	4.6	41.2	0.00	53.90	68.80	0.39
	1.00	c							
flour, white, unenriched	100.0	g	359	6.9	79.8	0.00	26.00	33.00	0.19
						0.00	53.30	67.60	0.39
white, steamed, Chinese restaurant	100.0	g	151	3.2	33.9				
cup, loosely packed	132.0	g	199	4.2	44.7	1.00	265.0	319.0	3.85
	1.00	c							
white, medium-grain, cooked	100.0	g	130	2.4	28.6	201.0	86.00	102.0	0.96
unenriched	186.0	g	242	4.4	53.2	394.0	169.0	200.0	1.88
	1.00	c							
white, short-grain, cooked	100.0	g	130	2.4	28.7	3.00	101.0	82.00	0.34
unenriched	205.0	g	266	4.8	58.8	4.92	166.0	134.0	0.56
	1.00	c							
flour, brown,	100.0	g	365	7.2	75.5	7.00	427.0	433.0	1.08
						11.20	683.0	693.0	1.73
brown, cooked, no salt, no fat	100.0	g	122	2.7	25.5				
	196.0	g	239	5.4	49.9	5.00	75.00	94.00	1.30
	1.00	c							
wild, cooked	100.0	g	101	4.0	21.3	5.00	20.00	33.00	0.27
	164.0	g	166	6.5	35.0	6.60	26.40	43.60	0.36
	1.00	c							
wild, raw	100.0	g	357	14.7	74.9	0.00	29.00	37.00	0.21
	160.0	g	571	23.6	120.0	0.00	53.90	68.80	0.39
	1.00	c							

OATS

	SERVING QUANTITY	SERVING UNIT	CALORIES (kCal)	PROTEIN (g)	TOTAL CARBOHYDRATES (g)	SODIUM (mg)	POTASSIUM (mg)	PHOSPHORUS (mg)	TOTAL FAT (g)
raw	100.0	g	379	12.2	67.7	6.00	362.0	410.0	6.52
	81.00	g	307	10.7	54.8	4.86	293.0	332.0	5.28
	1.00	c							
cereal, oat,	100.0	g	372	12.4	73.2	497.0	633.0	357.0	6.60
	33.00	g	123	4.1	24.2	164.0	209.0	118.0	2.18
	1.00	c							
steel cut	100.0	g	378	13.3	66.7	0.00	356.0	na	6.67
Brand: ARROWHEAD MILLS	45.00	g	170	6.0	30.0	0.00	160.0	na	3.00
	1.00	svg							
rolled	100.0	g	350	12.5	67.5	0.00	350.0	na	6.25
Brand: MILLVILLE by Aldi	40.00	g	140	5.0	27.0	0.00	140.0	na	2.50
	1.00	svg							
bran, cooked	100.0	g	40	3.2	11.4	1.00	92.00	119.0	0.86
	219.0	g	88	7.0	25.1	2.19	201.0	261.0	1.88
	1.00	c							
bran, uncooked (raw)	100.0	g	246	17.3	66.2	4.00	566.0	734.0	7.03
	94.00	g	231	16.3	62.2	3.76	532.0	690.0	6.61
	1.00	c							
flour, partially debranned	100.0	g	404	14.7	65.7	19.00	371.0	452.0	9.12
	104.0	g	420	15.2	68.3	19.80	386.0	470.0	9.48
	1.00	c							
regular, rolled, not fortified, dry	100.0	g	379	13.2	67.7	6.00	362.0	410.0	6.52
	81.00	g	307	10.7	54.8	4.86	293.0	332.0	5.28
	1.00	c							

WHEAT

	SERVING QUANTITY	SERVING UNIT	CALORIES (kcal)	PROTEIN (g)	TOTAL CARBOHYDRATES (g)	SODIUM (mg)	POTASSIUM (mg)	PHOSPHORUS (mg)	TOTAL FAT (g)
durum	100.0	g	399	13.7	71.1	2.00	431.0	508.0	2.47
	192.0	g	651	26.3	137	3.84	828.0	975.0	4.74
	1.00	c							
sprouted	100.0	g	198	7.5	42.5	16.00	169.0	200.0	1.27
	108.0	g	214	8.1	45.9	17.30	183.0	216.0	1.37
	1.00	c							
germ	100.0	g	360	23.2	51.8	12.00	892.0	842.0	9.72
	115.0	g	414	26.7	59.6	13.80	1,030	968	11.20
	1.00	c							
bran	100.0	g	216	15.6	64.5	2.00	1,180	1,010	4.25
	58.00	g	125	9.1	37.4	1.16	684.0	586.0	2.46
	1.00	c							
cream of wheat, instant, dry	100.0	g	366	10.6	75.5	571.0	115.0	103.0	1.40
	11.50	g	42	1.2	8.7	65.70	13.20	11.80	0.16
	1.00	tbsp							
flour, whole wheat, unenriched	100.0	g	370	15.1	71.2	3.00	376.0	352.0	2.73
whole grain, soft wheat	100.0	g	332	9.6	74.5	3.00	394.0	323.0	1.95
bread flour, unenriched	100.0	g	361	12.0	72.5	2.00	100.0	97.00	1.66
unsifted	137.0	g	495	16.4	99.4	2.74	137.0	133.0	2.27
	1.00	c							
flour, bread, white, enriched	100.0	g	361	12.0	72.5	2.00	100.0	97.00	1.66
	137.0	g	495	16.4	99.4	2.74	137.0	133.0	2.27
	1.00	c							
fllour, cake, enriched	100.0	g	362	8.2	78.0	2.00	105.0	85.00	0.86
unsifted	137.0	g	496	11.2	107.0	2.74	144.0	116.0	1.18
	1.00	c							

CORN

CORN	SERVING QUANTITY	SERVING UNIT	CALORIES (Kcal)	PROTEIN (g)	TOTAL CARBOHYDRATES (g)	SODIUM (mg)	POTASSIUM (mg)	PHOSPHORUS (mg)	TOTAL FAT (g)
white, sweet	100.0	g	390	7.8	86.6	956.0	88.00	39.00	
	25.00	g	98	2.0	21.7	239.0	22.00	9.75	
	1.00	c							
white, steamed (Navajo)	100.0	g	386	9.7	75.2	4.00	532.0	312.0	
	85.05	g	328	8.3	64.0	3.40	452.4	265.3	
	3.00	oz							
white, stew, steamed (Navajo)	100.0	g	112	8.8	10.8	104.0	177.0	107.0	
	85.05	g	95	7.5	9.2	88.45	150.5	91.00	
	3.00	oz							
sweet, boiled, drained	100.0	g	94	3.1	22.3	4.00	251.0	75.00	0.74
	82.00	g	77	2.6	18.3	3.28	205.8	61.50	0.61
	0.50	c							
flour, white, whole grain	100.0	g	361	6.9	76.9	5.00	315.0	272.0	3.86
	29.25	g	106	2.0	22.5	1.46	92.14	79.56	1.13
	0.25	c							
yellow, sweet, boiled, drained	100.0	g	96	3.4	21.0	1.00	218.0	77.00	1.50
	82.00	g	79	2.8	17.2	0.82	178.7	63.14	1.23
	0.50	c							
yellow, sweet, on the cob	100.0	g	86	3.3	18.7	15.00	270.0	89.00	1.35
	154.0	g	77	2.9	16.8	13.50	243.0	80.10	1.22
	1.00	c							
yello, sweet, creamed, canned	100.0	g	72	1.7	18.1	261.0	134.0	51.00	0.42
	128.0	g	92	2.2	23.2	334.1	171.5	65.28	0.54
	0.50	c							
yellow, sweet, kernels, frozen	100.0	g	88	3.0	20.7	3.00	213.0	70.00	0.78
	82.00	g	72	2.5	17.0	2.46	174.6	57.40	0.64
	0.50	c							
yellow, sweet, canned with liquid	100.0	g	61	2.0	13.9	195.0	136.0	46.00	0.77
	128.0	g	78	2.5	17.7	249.6	174.1	58.88	0.99
	0.50	c							
tortilla, no salt added	100.0	g	222	5.7	46.6	11.00	154.0	314.0	2.50
	26.00	g	58	1.5	12.1	2.86	40.04	81.64	0.65
	1.00	pc							

35

QUINOA	SERVING QUANTITY	SERVING UNIT	CALORIES (kCal)	PROTEIN (g)	TOTAL CARBOHYDRATES (g)	SODIUM (mg)	POTASSIUM (mg)	PHOSPHORUS (mg)	TOTAL FAT (g)
cooked	100.0	g	120	4.4	21.3	7.00	172.0	152.0	1.92
	185.0	g	222	8.1	39.4	13.00	318.0	281.0	3.55
	1.00	c							
uncooked	100.0	g	368	14.1	64.2	5.00	563.0	457.0	6.07
	170.0	g	626	24.0	109	8.50	957.0	777.0	10.30
	1.00	c							
pasta from quinoa flour (gluten-free)	100.0	g	152	3.2	31.1	4.00	63.00	91.00	2.07
	132.0	g	201	4.3	41.1	5.28	83.20	120.0	2.73
not packed	1.00	c							

D. PROTEINS

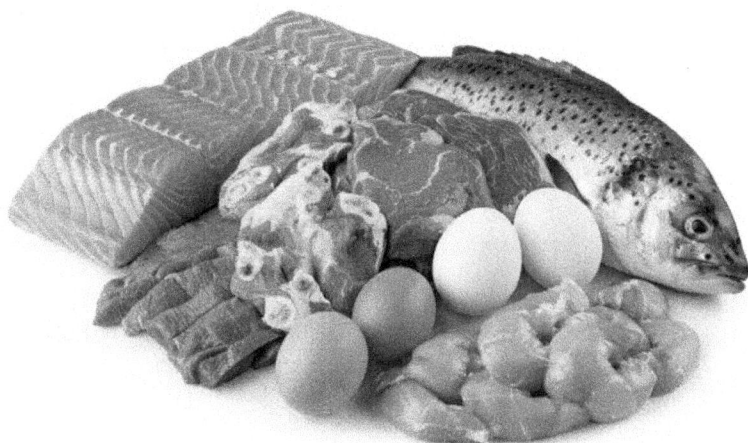

BEEF	SERVING QUANTITY	SERVING UNIT	CALORIES (kCal)	PROTEIN (g)	TOTAL CARBOHYDRATES (g)	SODIUM (mg)	POTASSIUM (mg)	PHOSPHORUS (mg)	TOTAL FAT (g)
chuck eyeroast, boneless, all grades 0" fat, separable lean only, **roasted**	3 85.05 3.00	g g oz	183 156	26.7 22.7	0.0 0.0	68.04 80.00	344.0 292.5	210.0 178.6	8.46 7.20
chuck eyeroast, boneless, all grades separable lean only, 0", **raw**	100.00 85.05 3.00	g g oz	137 117	20.6 17.5	0.0 0.0	85.00 72.29	357.0 303.6	204.0 173.5	6.01 5.11
chuck eyeroast, boneless, all grades sep lean & fat, 0" fat, **roasted**	100.00 85.05 3.00	g g oz	236 201	24.6 21.0	0.0 0.0	76.00 64.64	308.0 261.9	187.0 159.0	15.29 13.00
chuck eyeroast, boneless, all grades sep lean & fat, 0" fat, **raw**	100.0 85.05 3.00	g g oz	173 147	19.3 16.4	0.0 0.0	82.00 69.74	367.0 312.1	187.0 159.0	10.67 9.07
jerky	100.0 28.35 1.00	g g oz	410 116	33.2 9.4	11 3.1	1,785 506.05	597.0 169.2	407.0 115.3	25.60 7.26
corned beef, brisket, **raw**	100.0 113.4 4.00	g g oz	198 225	14.7 16.7	0.1 0.2	1,217 1,380	297.0 336.8	117.0 132.6	14.90 16.90
corned beef, brisket, **cooked**	100.0 85.05 3.00	g g oz	251 213	18.2 15.5	0.5 0.4	927.99 827.53	145.0 123.3	125.0 106.3	18.98 16.14
broth cube 1 cube, 6 fl. oz prepared	100.0 3.60 1.00	g g cube	170 6	17.3 0.6	16 0.6	24,000 864.00	403.0 14.51	225.0 8.10	4.00 0.14
liver, pan fried	100.0 81.00 1.00	g g slice	175 142	26.5 21.5	5.2 4.2	77.00 62.37	351.0 284.3	485.0 392.8	4.68 3.79
liver, braised	100.0 85.05 3.00	g g oz	191 162	29.1 24.7	5.1 4.4	79.00 67.19	352.0 299.3	496.9 422.6	5.26 4.47
tongue, simmered	100.0 85.05 3.00	g g oz	284 242	19.3 16.4	0.0 0.0	65.00 55.28	184.0 156.5	145.0 123.3	22.30 18.97
kidney simmered	100.0 85.05 3.00	g g oz	158 134	27.3 23.2	0.0 0.0	94.00 79.95	135.0 114.8	304.0 258.5	4.65 3.95
tripe, simmered	100.0 85.05 3.00	g g oz	94 80	11.7 10.0	2.0 1.7	68.00 57.83	42.00 35.72	66.00 56.13	4.05 3.44

CHICKEN

	SERVING QUANTITY	SERVING UNIT	CALORIES (kCal)	PROTEIN (g)	TOTAL CARBOHYDRATES (g)	SODIUM (mg)	POTASSIUM (mg)	PHOSPHORUS (mg)	TOTAL FAT (g)
ground, raw	100.0	g	143	17.4	0.0	60.00	522.0	178.0	8.10
meat and skin,	100.0	g	215	18.6	0.0	70.00	189.0	147.0	15.06
raw	113.4	g	244	21.1	0.0	79.38	214.3	166.7	17.08
	4.00	oz							
meat and skin,	100.0	g	239	27.3	0.0	82.00	223.0	182.0	13.60
roasted	85.05	g	203	23.2	0.0	69.74	189.6	154.7	11.57
	3.00	oz							
thigh meat	100.0	g	218	28.2	1.2	95.00	259.0	199.0	10.30
only, fried	85.05	g	185	24.0	1.0	80.80	220.2	169.2	8.76
	3.00	oz							
thigh meat	100.0	g	179	24.8	0.0	106.0	269.0	230.0	8.15
only, roasted	85.05	g	152	21.1	0.0	90.15	228.7	195.6	6.93
	3.00	oz							
wing meat only,	100.0	g	211	30.2	0.0	91.00	208.0	164.0	9.15
fried	85.05	g	179	25.6	0.0	77.39	176.9	139.4	7.78
	3.00	oz							
wing meat only,	100.0	g	203	30.5	0.0	92.00	210.0	166.0	8.13
roasted	85.05	g	173	26.0	0.0	78.25	178.6	141.1	6.91
	3.00	oz							
wing meat only,	100.0	g	181	27.2	0.0	73.00	153.0	134.0	7.18
stewed	85.05	g	154	23.1	0.0	62.09	130.1	113.9	6.11
	3.00	oz							
back meat only,	100.0	g	288	30.0	5.7	99.00	251.0	176.0	4.12
fried	85.05	g	245	25.5	4.8	84.20	213.4	149.6	3.50
	3.00	oz							
back meat only,	100.0	g	239	28.2	0.0	96.00	237.0	165.0	13.16
roasted	85.05	g	203	24.0	0.0	81.65	201.5	140.3	11.19
	3.00	oz							
back meat only,	100.0	g	209	25.3	0.0	67.00	158.0	130.0	11.19
stewed	85.05	g	178	21.5	0.0	56.98	134.3	110.5	9.52
	3.00	oz							
drumstick meat	100.0	g	195	28.6	0.0	96.00	249.0	186.0	8.08
only, fried	85.05	g	166	24.3	0.0	81.65	211.7	158.1	6.87
	3.00	oz							
drumstick meat	100.0	g	155	24.2	0.0	128.0	256.0	200.0	5.70
only, roasted	85.05	g	132	20.6	0.0	108.8	217.7	170.1	4.85
	3	oz							

CHICKEN

CHICKEN	SERVING QUANTITY	SERVING UNIT	CALORIES (kcal)	PROTEIN (g)	TOTAL CARBOHYDRATES (g)	SODIUM (mg)	POTASSIUM (mg)	PHOSPHORUS (mg)	TOTAL FAT (g)
drumstick meat only, stewed	100.0	g	169	27.5	0.0	80.00	199.0	150.0	5.71
	85.05 3.00	g oz	144	23.4	0.0	68.04	169.2	127.5	4.86
leg meat only, fried	100.0	g	208	28.4	0.7	96.00	254.0	193.0	9.32
	85.05 3.00	g oz	177	24.1	0.6	81.65	216.0	164.1	7.93
leg meat only, roasted	100.0	g	174	24.2	0.0	99.00	269.0	205.0	7.80
	85.05 3.00	g oz	148	20.6	0.0	84.20	228.7	174.3	6.63
leg meat only, stewed	100.0	g	185	26.3	0.0	78.00	190.0	149.0	8.06
	85.05 3.00	g oz	157	22.3	0.0	66.34	161.6	126.7	6.85
pate, chicken liver, canned	100.0	g	201	13.5	6.6	386.0	95.00	175.0	13.10
	52.00 4.00	g tbsp	105	7.0	3.4	200.7	49.40	91.00	6.81
chicken tenders, fast food	100.0	g	271	19.2	17.3	769.0	373.0	282.0	13.95
	62.00 4.00	g pcs	168	11.9	10.7	476.8	231.2	174.8	8.65
chicken patty, frozen, cooked	100.0	g	287	14.9	12.8	532.0	261.0	208.0	19.58
bratwurst, chicken, cooked	100.0	g	176	19.4	0.0	72.00	211.0	160.0	10.30
	83.92 2.96	g oz	148	16.3	0.0	60.42	177.0	134.2	8.69
sausage, chicken/beef, smoked	100.0	g	295	18.5	0.0	1,020	139.0	111.0	244.0
	138.0 1.00	g c	251	15.7	0.0	867.5	118.2	94.41	20.41

TURKEY	SERVING QUANTITY	SERVING UNIT	CALORIES (kcal)	PROTEIN (g)	TOTAL CARBOHYDRATES (g)	SODIUM (mg)	POTASSIUM (mg)	PHOSPHORUS (mg)	TOTAL FAT (g)
breast, meat & skin, raw	100.0	g	144	21.6	0.1	112.0	224.0	183.0	5.64
	113.4	g	163	24.5	0.2	127.0	254.0	207.5	6.40
	4.00	oz							
breast, meat & skin, roasted	100.0	g	189	28.6	0.1	103.0	239.0	223.0	7.39
	85.05	g	161	24.3	0.1	87.60	203.2	189.6	6.29
	3.00	oz							
breast, meat only, raw	100.0	g	114	23.3	0.0	74.00	267.0	185.0	2.33
	85.05	g	97	19.9	0.0	62.94	227.0	157.3	1.98
	3.00	oz							
breast, meat only, roasted	100.0	g	136	29.5	0.0	114.0	297.0	253.0	1.97
	85.05	g	116	25.1	0.0	96.96	252.6	215.1	1.68
	3.00	oz							
ground, raw	100.0	g	148	20.0	0.0	58.00	237.0	200.0	7.66
	113.4	g	168	22.3	0.0	65.77	268.7	226.8	8.69
	4.00	oz							
ground, cooked	100.0	g	203	27.4	0.0	78.00	294.0	254.0	10.40
	85.05	g	173	23.3	0.0	66.34	250.0	216.0	8.85
	3.00	oz							
white rotisserie, deli cut	100.0	g	112	13.5	7.7	1,200	349.0	158.0	3.00
	56.70	g	64	7.7	4.4	680.4	197.8	89.59	1.70
	2.00	oz							
ham, extra lean, sliced	100.0	g	134	19.6	0.9	1,038	299.0	304.0	5.80
	20.00	g	27	3.9	0.2	207.6	59.80	60.80	1.16
	1.00	pc							
pastrami, sliced	100.0	g	139	16.3	3.3	1,123	345.0	200.0	6.21
	56.70	g	79	9.2	1.9	636.7	195.6	113.4	3.52
	2.00	slices							
bologna	100.0	g	209	11.4	4.7	1,071	135.0	114.0	16.05
	56.70	g	119	6.5	2.7	607.2	76.55	64.64	9.10
	2.00	slices							
salami	100.0	g	172	19.2	1.6	1,107	216.0	266.0	9.21
	56.70	g	98	10.9	0.9	627.6	122.4	150.8	5.22
	2.00	slices							
bacon, turkey, cooked	100.0	g	382	29.6	3.1	2,285	395.0	460.0	27.90
	28.35	g	108	8.4	0.9	647.8	111.9	130.4	7.91
	1.00	oz							
bacon, turkey, low sodium	100.0	g	253	13.3	4.8	900.0	156.0	145.0	20.00
	15.00	g	38	2.0	0.7	135.0	23.40	21.75	3.00
	1.00	svg							
sausage, turkey, cooked	100.0	g	196	23.9	0.0	665.0	298.0	202.0	10.44
	56.70	g	111	13.6	0.0	377.0	168.9	114.5	5.92
	2.00	oz							

EGG	SERVING QUANTITY	SERVING UNIT	CALORIES (kcal)	PROTEIN (g)	TOTAL CARBOHYDRATES (g)	SODIUM (mg)	POTASSIUM (mg)	PHOSPHORUS (mg)	TOTAL FAT (g)
chicken, raw,	100.0	g	143	12.6	0.7	142.0	138.0	198.0	9.51
large	50.00	g	72	6.3	0.4	71.00	69.00	99.00	4.76
	1.00	pc							
chicken, fried,	100.0	g	196	13.6	0.8	207.0	152.0	215.0	14.84
large	46.00	g	90	6.3	0.4	95.22	69.92	98.90	6.83
	1.00	pc							
chicken, poached,	100.0	g	143	12.5	0.7	297.0	138.0	197.0	9.47
large	50.00	g	72	6.3	0.4	148.5	69.00	98.50	4.74
	1.00	pc							
chicken, hard	100.0	g	155	12.6	1.1	124.0	126.0	172.0	10.61
boiled, large	50.00	g	78	6.3	0.6	62.00	63.00	86.00	5.31
	1.00	pc							
scrambled, fast	100.0	g	212	13.8	2.1	187.0	147.0	242.0	16.18
food	94.00	g	199	13.0	2.0	175.7	138.1	227.4	15.21
	2.00	pc							
substitute, liquid	100.0	g	84	12.0	0.6	177.0	330.0	121.0	3.31
	251.0	g	211	30.1	1.6	444.2	828.3	303.7	8.31
	1.00	c							
substitute,	100.0	g	443	55.8	22	798.2	742.3	476.9	12.97
powder	9.92	g	44	5.5	2.2	79.20	73.66	47.32	1.29
	0.35	oz							
substitute, frozen	100.0	g	160	11.3	3.2	199.0	213.0	72.00	11.11
	60.00	g	96	6.8	1.9	119.4	127.8	43.20	6.67
	0.25	c							
chicken, egg	100.0	g	52	10.9	0.7	166.0	163.0	15.00	0.17
whites only, raw	33.00	g	17	3.6	0.2	54.78	53.79	4.95	0.06
large egg	1.00	pc							
chicken, yolk	100.0	g	322	15.9	3.6	48.00	109.0	390.0	26.54
only, raw	17.00	g	55	2.7	0.6	8.16	18.53	66.30	4.51
large egg	1.00	pc							
chicken, whole,	100.0	g	147	12.3	1.0	128.0	135.0	193.0	9.95
raw, frozen	56.70	g	83	7.0	0.6	72.57	76.54	109.4	5.64
	2.00	oz							
yolk only, frozen,	100.0	g	296	15.5	0.8	67.00	121.0	419.9	25.60
raw	56.70	g	168	8.8	0.5	37.99	68.61	238.1	14.51
	2.00	oz							
whites, frozen,	100.0	g	48	10.2	1.0	169.0	169.0	13.00	0.00
raw	56.70	g	27	5.8	0.6	95.82	95.82	7.37	0.00
	2.00	oz							
duck, raw	100.0	g	185	12.8	1.5	146.0	222.0	220.0	13.77
	70.00	g	130	9.0	1.0	102.2	155.4	154.0	9.64
	1.00	pc							
quail, raw	100.0	g	158	13.1	0.4	141.0	132.0	226.0	11.09
	9.00	g	14	1.2	0.0	12.69	11.88	20.34	1.00
	1.00	pc							

TOFU	SERVING QUANTITY	SERVING UNIT	CALORIES (kCal)	PROTEIN (g)	TOTAL CARBOHYDRATES (g)	SODIUM (mg)	POTASSIUM (mg)	PHOSPHORUS (mg)	TOTAL FAT (g)
soft with calcium	100.00	g	61	7.2	1.2	8.00	120.00	92.00	3.69
sulfate and	85.05	g	52	6.1	1.0	6.80	102.06	78.25	3.14
magnesium chloride (Nigari)	3.00	oz							
firm with calcium	100.00	g	78	9.0	2.9	12.00	148.00	121.00	4.17
sulfate and magnesium	85.05	g	66	7.7	2.4	10.21	125.87	102.91	3.55
chloride (Nigari)									
	3.00	oz							
silken tofu	100.00	g	43	4.8	0.6	2.00	na	na	2.40
(Vitasoy USA)	91.00	g	39	4.4	0.5	1.82	na	na	2.18
	0.20	package							
SALMON									
pink, raw	100.00	g	127	20.5	0.0	74.99	365.96	260.98	4.40
	113.40	g	144	23.2	0.0	85.04	415.00	295.95	4.99
	4.00	oz							
atlantic, wild, raw	100.00	g	142	19.8	0.0	44.00	489.95	199.98	0.98
	113.40	g	161	22.5	0.0	49.89	555.61	226.78	1.11
	4.00	oz							
atlantic,	100.00	g	208	20.4	0.0	58.99	362.97	239.98	13.42
farmed, raw	113.39	g	236	23.2	0.0	66.90	411.60	272.13	15.22
	4.00	oz							
pink, canned, drained	100.00	g	138	23.1	0.0	380.78	332.80	378.78	5.02
solids, w/ bone	85.05	g	117	19.6	0.0	323.85	283.05	322.15	4.27
	3.00	oz							
	100.00	g	139	19.8	0.0	75.00	325.99	328.99	6.05
pink, canned, with	56.70	g	79	11.2	0.0	42.52	184.84	186.54	3.43
bone and liquid no salt	2.00	oz							
pink, canned, drained	100.00	g	136	24.6	0.0	378.00	326.00	253.00	4.21
solids	85.05	g	116	20.9	0.0	321.49	277.26	215.18	3.58
without skin and bones	3.00	oz							
chum, canned,	100.00	g	141	21.4	0.0	75.00	300.00	353.99	5.50
drained, with bone	56.70	g	80	12.2	0.0	42.52	170.10	200.71	3.12
no salt	2.00	oz							
nuggets, breaded,	100.00	g	212	12.7	14	173.00	165.00	176.00	11.72
frozen, heated									
TILAPIA									
raw	100.00	g	96	20.1	0.0	52.00	302.0	170.0	1.70
	113.40	g	107	22.8	0.0	58.97	342.5	192.8	1.93
	4.00	oz							
cooked, dry heat	100.00	g	128	26.2	0.0	55.97	379.8	203.9	2.65
	85.05	g	109	22.2	0.0	47.60	323.0	173.4	2.25
	3.00	oz							

	SERVING QUANTITY	SERVING UNIT	CALORIES (kcal)	PROTEIN (g)	TOTAL CARBOHYDRATES (g)	SODIUM (mg)	POTASSIUM (mg)	PHOSPHORUS (mg)	TOTAL FAT (g)
SARDINES									
spanish	100.0	g	212	6.2	14.2	310.00	0.00	na	14.16
	113.0	g	240	7.0	16.0	350.00	0.00	na	16.00
	4.00	oz							
atlantic, canned in oil, with bones	100.0	g	208	24.6	0.0	307.00	397.0	490.0	11.45
	24.00	g	50	5.9	0.0	73.68	95.28	117.6	2.75
	2.00	oz							
portuguese	100.0	g	236	25.5	0.0	500.00	na	na	12.73
	55.00	g	130	14.0	0.0	275.00	na	na	7.00
	0.50	c							
fillets, canned	100.0	g	338	18.2	7.3	364.00	na	na	26.36
	55.00	g	186	10.0	4.0	200.00	na	na	14.50
	0.25	c							
TUNA									
bluefin, raw	100.0	g	144	23.3	0.0	39.00	251.9	253.9	4.90
	113.4	g	163	26.5	0.0	44.22	285.7	288.0	5.56
	4.00	oz							
yellowfin or Ahi, raw	100.0	g	109	24.4	0.0	45.00	440.9	277.9	0.49
	113.4	g	124	27.7	0.0	51.03	500.0	315.2	0.56
	4.00	oz							
canned in oil, drained, light no salt	100.0	g	198	29.1	0.0	50.00	207.0	311.0	8.21
	56.70	g	112	16.5	0.0	28.35	117.3	176.3	4.65
	2.00	oz							
white, canned in water, drained no salt	100.0	g	128	23.6	0.0	50.00	237.0	217.0	2.97
	56.70	g	73	13.4	0.0	28.35	134.3	123.0	1.68
	2.00	oz							
canned in water, drained, light no salt	100.0	g	116	25.5	0.0	50.00	237.0	163.0	0.82
	56.70	g	66	14.5	0.0	28.35	134.3	92.42	0.46
	2.00	oz							
white, canned in oil, drained, no salt	100.0	g	186	26.5	0.0	50.00	332.9	267.0	8.08
	56.70	g	105	15.0	0.0	28.35	188.8	151.3	4.58
	2.00	oz							

TROUT

	SERVING QUANTITY	SERVING UNIT	CALORIES (kCal)	PROTEIN (g)	TOTAL CARBOHYDRATES (g)	SODIUM (mg)	POTASSIUM (mg)	PHOSPHORUS (mg)	TOTAL FAT (g)
rainbow, wild, raw, fillet	100.0	g	119	20.5	0.0	31.00	481.0	271.0	3.46
	113.4	g	135	23.2	0.0	35.15	545.4	307.3	3.92
	4.00	oz							
rainbow, farmed, raw, fillet	100.0	g	141	19.9	0.0	51.00	376.9	225.9	6.18
	113.4	g	160	22.6	0.0	57.83	427.4	256.2	7.01
	4.00	oz							
mixed species, raw fillet	100.0	g	148	20.8	0.0	52.00	360.9	244.9	6.61
	113.4	g	168	23.6	0.0	58.96	409.3	277.8	7.50
	4.00	oz							
sea trout, mixed species, raw	100.0	g	104	16.7	0.0	57.99	340.9	249.9	3.61
	113.4	g	118	19.0	0.0	65.77	386.6	283.4	4.09
	4.00	oz							
rainbow, wild, cooked, dry heat	100.0	g	150	22.9	0.0	56.00	448.0	269.0	5.82
	85.05	g	128	19.5	0.0	47.63	381.0	228.7	4.95
	3.00	oz							
rainbow, farmed, cooked, dry heat	100.0	g	168	23.8	0.0	61.00	450.0	270.0	7.38
	85.05	g	143	20.2	0.0	51.88	382.7	229.6	6.28
	3.00	oz							
mixed species, cooked, dry heat	100.0	g	190	26.6	0.0	67.00	463.0	314.0	8.47
	85.05	g	162	22.7	0.0	56.98	393.7	267.0	7.20
	3.00	oz							
sea trout, mixed species, cooked, dry heat	100.0	g	133	21.5	0.0	74.00	437.0	321.0	4.63
	85.05	g	113	18.3	0.0	62.94	371.6	273.0	3.94
	3.00	oz							

HALIBUT

	SERVING QUANTITY	SERVING UNIT	CALORIES (kCal)	PROTEIN (g)	TOTAL CARBOHYDRATES (g)	SODIUM (mg)	POTASSIUM (mg)	PHOSPHORUS (mg)	TOTAL FAT (g)
greenland, raw	100.0	g	186	14.4	0.0	79.99	267.9	163.9	13.84
	113.4	g	211	16.3	0.0	90.71	303.8	185.9	15.69
	4.00	oz							
atlantic and pacific, raw	100.0	g	91	18.6	0.0	67.99	434.9	235.9	1.33
	113.4	g	103	21.0	0.0	77.10	493.2	267.6	1.51
	4.00	oz							
greenland, cooked, dry heat	100.0	g	239	18.4	0.0	103.0	344.0	210.0	17.7
	85.05	g	203	15.7	0.0	87.60	292.5	178.6	15.09
	3.00	oz							
atlantic and pacific, cooked, dry heat	100.0	g	111	22.5	0.0	82.00	527.9	287.0	1.61
	85.05	g	94	19.2	0.0	69.74	449.0	244.1	1.37
	3.00	oz							

COD	SERVING QUANTITY	SERVING UNIT	CALORIES (Kcal)	PROTEIN (g)	TOTAL CARBOHYDRATES (g)	SODIUM (mg)	POTASSIUM (mg)	PHOSPHORUS (mg)	TOTAL FAT (g)
atlantic, raw	100.0	g	82	17.8	0.0	54.00	412.9	202.9	0.67
	113.4	g	93	20.2	0.0	61.23	468.3	230.1	0.76
	4.00	oz							
atlantic, canned	100.0	g	105	22.8	0.0	218.0	527.9	260.0	0.86
	56.70	g	60	12.9	0.0	123.6	299.3	147.4	0.49
	2.00	oz							
atlantic, cooked,	100.0	g	105	22.8	0.0	78.00	244.0	138.0	0.86
dry heat	85.05	g	89	19.4	0.0	66.34	207.5	117.3	0.73
	3.00	oz							
pacific, raw	100.0	g	69	15.3	0.0	302.9	234.9	280.9	0.41
	113.4	g	78	17.3	0.0	343.5	266.4	318.6	0.46
	4.00	oz							
pacific, cooked, dry	100.0	g	85	18.7	0.0	372.0	289.0	345.0	0.50
heat	85.05	g	72	15.9	0.0	316.3	245.7	293.4	0.43
	3.00	oz							
LOBSTER									
Northern, raw (Langoustine)	100.0	g	77	16.5	0.0	423.0	200.0	161.0	0.75
	113.4	g	87	18.7	0.0	479.6	226.8	182.5	0.85
	4.00	oz							
Spiny, mixed species, raw	100.0	g	112	20.6	2.4	177.0	180.0	238.0	1.51
	113.4	g	127	23.4	2.8	200.7	104.1	269.8	1.71
	4.00	oz							
Northern, cooked, moist heat (Langoustine)	100.0	g	89	19.0	0.0	485.9	230.0	185.0	0.86
	85.05	g	76	16.2	0.0	413.3	195.6	157.3	0.73
	3.00	oz							
Spiny, mixed species, cooked, moist heat	100.0	g	143	26.4	3.1	227.0	208.0	229.0	1.94
	85.05	g	122	22.5	2.7	193.0	176.9	194.7	1.65
	3.00	oz							

CRAB

	SERVING QUANTITY	SERVING UNIT	CALORIES (KCal)	PROTEIN (g)	TOTAL CARBOHYDRATES (g)	SODIUM (mg)	POTASSIUM (mg)	PHOSPHORUS (mg)	TOTAL FAT (g)
blue, raw	100.0	g	87	18.1	0.0	293.00	329.00	229.00	1.08
	113.4	g	99	20.5	0.5	332.26	373.09	259.69	1.22
	4.00	oz							
blue, canned	100.0	g	83	17.9	0.0	562.99	259.00	234.00	0.74
	56.70	g	47	10.1	0.0	319.22	146.85	132.68	0.42
	2.00	oz							
dungeness, raw	100.0	g	86	17.4	0.7	295.00	354.00	182.00	0.97
	113.4	g	98	19.7	0.8	334.53	401.44	206.39	1.10
	4.00	oz							
dungeness, cooked, moist heat	100.0	g	110	22.3	1.0	378.00	408.00	175.00	1.24
	85.05	g	94	19.0	0.8	321.49	347.00	148.84	1.05
	3.00	oz							
alaska king, raw	100.0	g	84	18.3	0.0	836.00	204.00	219.00	0.60
	113.4	g	95	20.7	0.0	948.02	231.34	248.35	0.68
	4.00	oz							
alaska king, cooked, moist heat	100.0	g	97	19.4	0.0	1,072	262.00	280.00	1.54
	85.05	g	83	16.5	0.0	911.73	222.83	238.14	1.31
	3.00	oz							
imitation, crabmeat (Kani)	100.0	g	95	7.6	15.0	528.99	90.00	282.00	0.46
	85.05	g	81	6.5	12.8	449.91	76.54	239.84	0.39
	3.00	oz							
cakes	100.0	g	266	18.8	8.5	819.00	270.00	378.00	17.25
	60.00	g	160	11.3	5.1	491.00	162.00	226.80	10.35
	1.00	pc							

CATFISH

	SERVING QUANTITY	SERVING UNIT	CALORIES (KCal)	PROTEIN (g)	TOTAL CARBOHYDRATES (g)	SODIUM (mg)	POTASSIUM (mg)	PHOSPHORUS (mg)	TOTAL FAT (g)
channel, wild, raw	100.0	g	95	16.4	0.0	43.00	405.93	208.98	2.82
	113.4	g	108	18.6	0.0	48.76	357.97	236.98	3.20
	4.00	oz							
channel, farmed, raw	100.0	g	119	15.2	0.0	97.94	301.82	203.88	5.94
	85.05	g	101	13.0	0.0	83.30	256.70	173.40	5.05
	3.00	oz							
breaded, fried	100.0	g	229	18.1	8.0	280.00	340.00	216.00	13.33
	85.05	g	195	15.4	6.8	238.14	289.17	183.71	11.34
	3.00	oz							
wild, cooked, dry heat	100.0	g	105	18.5	0.0	50.00	419.00	304.00	2.85
	85.05	g	89	15.7	0.0	42.52	356.36	258.55	2.42
	3.00	oz							
farmed, cooked, dry heat	100.0	g	144	18.4	0.0	119.00	366.00	247.00	7.19
	85.05	g	122	15.7	0.0	101.21	311.28	210.07	6.12
	3.00	oz							

MUSSELS

	SERVING QUANTITY	SERVING UNIT	CALORIES (kCal)	PROTEIN (g)	TOTAL CARBOHYDRATES (g)	SODIUM (mg)	POTASSIUM (mg)	PHOSPHORUS (mg)	TOTAL FAT (g)
blue, raw	100.0	g	86	11.9	3.7	286.00	320.00	197.00	2.24
	113.4	g	98	13.5	4.2	324.32	362.88	223.40	2.54
	4.00	oz							
blue, cooked,	100.0	g	172	23.8	7.4	369.00	268.00	285.00	4.48
moist heat	85.05	g	146	20.2	6.3	313.83	227.93	242.39	3.81
	3.00	oz							
atlantic or	100.0	g	197	8.8	11.6	415.25	243.87	159.06	12.56
pacific, meat only	85.05	g	167	7.5	9.9	353.17	207.41	1,315	10.69
	3.00	oz							

MACKEREL

	SERVING QUANTITY	SERVING UNIT	CALORIES (kCal)	PROTEIN (g)	TOTAL CARBOHYDRATES (g)	SODIUM (mg)	POTASSIUM (mg)	PHOSPHORUS (mg)	TOTAL FAT (g)
Atlantic or	100.0	g	205	18.6	0.0	89.99	313.97	216.98	13.89
Boston, raw fillet	113.4	g	232	21.1	0.0	102.05	356.04	246.05	15.75
	4.00	oz							
pacific and Jack,	100.0	g	158	20.1	0.0	85.99	405.96	124.99	7.89
raw fillet	113.4	g	179	22.8	0.0	97.51	460.36	141.71	8.95
	4.00	oz							
Atlantic Spanish, raw fillet	100.0	g	139	19.3	0.0	58.99	445.96	204.98	6.30
	113.4	g	158	21.9	0.0	66.90	505.71	232.45	7.14
	4.00	oz							
Jack, canned,	100.0	g	156	23.2	0.0	378.99	194.00	301.00	6.30
solids, drained	56.70	g	88	13.2	0.0	214.89	110.00	170.66	3.57
	2.00	oz							
Atlantic or	100.0	g	262	23.9	0.0	83.00	401.00	278.00	17.81
Boston, cooked, dry heat	85.05	g	223	20.3	0.0	70.59	341.05	236.44	15.15
	3.00	oz							
Atlantic, Spanish,	100.0	g	158	23.6	0.0	66.00	553.99	271.00	6.32
cooked, dry heat	85.05	g	134	20.1	0.0	56.13	471.17	230.48	5.38
	3.00	oz							
Pacific and Jack,	100.0	g	201	25.7	0.0	110.00	520.99	160.00	10.12
mixed species, cooked	85.05	g	171	21.9	0.0	93.55	443.11	136.08	8.61
	3.00	oz							

CLAMS

	SERVING QUANTITY	SERVING UNIT	CALORIES (kCal)	PROTEIN (g)	TOTAL CARBOHYDRATES (g)	SODIUM (mg)	POTASSIUM (mg)	PHOSPHORUS (mg)	TOTAL FAT (g)
mixed species, raw	100	g	86	14.7	3.6	601.00	46.00	198.00	0.96
	85.05	g	73	12.5	3.0	511.15	39.12	168.40	0.82
	3.00	oz							
mixed species, breaded, fried	100.0	g	202	14.2	10.3	364.00	326.00	188.00	11.15
	85.05	g	172	12.1	8.8	309.58	277.26	159.89	9.48
	3.00	oz							
mixed species, canned, with liquid	100.0	g	2	0.4	0.1	215.00	149.00	114.00	0.02
	28.35	g	1	0.1	0.0	60.95	42.24	32.32	0.01
	1.00	oz							
mixed species, canned, drained	100.0	g	142	24.3	5.9	112.00	627.99	326.99	1.59
	56.70	g	81	13.8	3.4	63.50	356.07	185.41	0.90
	2.00	oz							

OYSTERS

	SERVING QUANTITY	SERVING UNIT	CALORIES (kCal)	PROTEIN (g)	TOTAL CARBOHYDRATES (g)	SODIUM (mg)	POTASSIUM (mg)	PHOSPHORUS (mg)	TOTAL FAT (g)
ostrich, raw	100.0	g	125	21.6	0.0	83.00	297.00	204.00	3.67
	85.05	g	106	18.3	0.0	70.59	252.60	173.50	3.12
	3.00	oz							
ostrich, cooked	100.0	g	159	28.8	0.0	81.00	409.00	281.00	3.97
	85.05	g	135	24.5	0.0	68.89	347.85	238.99	3.38
	3.00	oz							
pacific, raw	100.0	g	81	9.5	5.0	106.00	168.00	162.00	2.30
	113.4	g	92	10.7	5.6	120.20	190.51	183.71	2.61
	4.00	oz							
pacific, cooked, moist heat	100.0	g	163	18.9	9.9	212.00	302.00	243.00	4.60
	85.05	g	139	16.1	8.4	180.30	256.85	206.67	3.91
	3.00	oz							
eastern, canned	100.0	g	68	7.1	3.9	112.00	229.00	139.00	2.47
	56.70	g	39	4.0	2.2	63.50	129.84	78.81	1.40
	2.00	oz							
eastern, farmed, raw	100.0	g	59	5.2	5.5	178.00	124.00	93.00	1.55
	85.05	g	50	4.4	4.7	151.39	105.46	79.10	1.32
	3.00	oz							
eastern, wild, raw	100.0	g	51	5.7	2.7	85.00	156.00	97.00	1.71
	113.4	g	58	6.5	3.1	96.39	176.90	110.00	1.94
	4.00	oz							
eastern, wild, breaded, fried	100.0	g	199	8.8	11.6	417.00	244.00	159.00	12.58
	85.05	g	169	7.5	9.9	354.65	207.52	135.23	10.70
	3.00	oz							
battered, breaded, fried, fast food	100.0	g	265	9.0	28.7	486.99	131.00	141.00	12.90
	85.05	g	225	7.7	24.4	414.19	111.41	119.92	10.97
	3.00	oz							

	SERVING QUANTITY	SERVING UNIT	CALORIES (kcal)	PROTEIN (g)	TOTAL CARBOHYDRATES (g)	SODIUM (mg)	POTASSIUM (mg)	PHOSPHORUS (mg)	TOTAL FAT (g)
SCALLOPS									
Mixed species, raw	100.0	g	69	12.1	3.2	392.00	205.00	12.80	0.49
	113.4 4.00	g oz	78	13.7	3.6	444.53	232.47	14.52	0.56
Bay and Sea, steamed	100.0	g	111	20.5	5.4	667.00	314.00	426.00	0.84
	85.05 3.00	g oz	94	17.5	4.6	567.28	267.06	362.31	0.71
mixed species, breaded and fried	100.0	g	216	18.1	10.1	464.00	333.00	236.00	10.94
	46.50 3.00	g pcs	100	8.4	4.7	215.76	15.85	109.74	5.09
breaded, fried, fast food	100.0	g	268	10.9	26.7	637.99	204.00	203.00	13.47
	85.05 3.00	g oz	228	9.3	22.7	542.61	173.50	172.65	11.46
SHRIMPS									
mixed species, raw	100.0	g	71	13.6	0.9	566.00	113.00	244.00	1.01
	113.4 4.00	g oz	81	15.4	1.0	641.84	128.14	276.40	1.15
mixed species, breaded, fried	100.0	g	242	21.4	12	343.80	224.87	217.87	12.27
	85.05 3.00	g oz	206	18.2	9.8	292.40	191.25	185.30	10.44
mixed species, cooked, moist heat	100.0	g	119	22.8	1.5	946.99	170.00	306.00	1.70
	85.05 3.00	g oz	101	19.4	1.3	805.41	144.58	260.25	1.45
cracker	100.0	g	426	7.1	59	571.00	193.00	191.00	17.86

E. DAIRY and DAIRY ALTERNATIVES

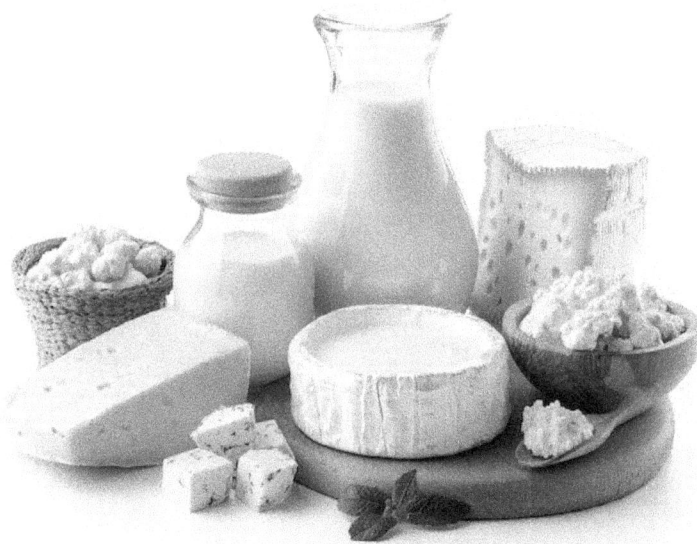

ALMOND	SERVING QUANTITY	SERVING UNIT	CALORIES (kcal)	PROTEIN (g)	TOTAL CARBOHYDRATES (g)	SODIUM (mg)	POTASSIUM (mg)	PHOSPHORUS (mg)	TOTAL FAT (g)
whole	100	g	579	21.2	21.6	1.00	733.0	481.0	49.9
	35.75	g	207	7.6	7.7	0.36	262.0	171.1	17.9
	0.25	c							
slivered	100	g	579	21.2	21.6	1.00	733.0	481.0	49.9
	27	g	156	5.7	5.8	0.27	197.9	129.9	13.5
	0.25	c							
ground	100	g	579	21.2	21.6	1.00	733.0	481.0	49.9
	23.75	g	138	5.0	5.1	0.24	174.1	114.4	11.9
	0.25	c							
paste (marzipan)	100	g	458	9.0	47.8	9.00	314.0	258.0	27.7
	28.38	g	130	2.6	13.6	2.55	89.10	73.21	7.9
	2	tbsp							
oil	100	g	884	0.0	0.0	0.00	0.00	0.00	100.0
	13.6	g	120	0.0	0.0	0.00	0.00	0.00	13.6
	1	tbsp							
butter, without salt added	100	g	614	21.0	18.8	227.0	748.0	508.0	55.5
	16	g	98	3.4	3.0	1.12	119.6	81.28	8.9
	1	tbsp							
dry roasted, without salt added	100	g	598	3.0	21.0	3.00	713.0	471.0	52.5
	34.5	g	206	7.2	7.3	1.04	245.1	162.50	18.1
	0.25	c							
oil roasted, without salt	100	g	607	21.2	17.7	1.00	699.0	466.0	55.2
	39.25	g	238	8.3	6.9	0.39	274.3	182.91	21.7
	0.25	c							
milk, unsweetened, shelf stable	100	g	15	0.4	1.3	72.00	67.00	9.00	1.0
	262	g	39	1.1	3.4	188.6	175.5	23.58	2.5
	1	c							
milk, sweetened, vanilla flavor ready-to-drink	100	g	38	0.4	6.6	63.00	50.00	8.00	1.0
	240	g	91	1.0	15.8	151.2	120.0	19.20	2.5
	1	c							
milk, chocolate flavor, unsweetened fortified Vit. D2 and E	100	g	21	0.8	1.3	75.00	96.00	17.00	1.5
	240	g	50	2.0	3.0	180.0	130.4	40.80	3.5
	1	c							

YOGURT

YOGURT	SERVING QUANTITY	SERVING UNIT	CALORIES (kcal)	PROTEIN (g)	TOTAL CARBOHYDRATES (g)	SODIUM (mg)	POTASSIUM (mg)	PHOSPHORUS (mg)	TOTAL FAT (g)
whole milk, flavored (non-fruit)	100	g	77	3.3	9.4	44.0	147.0	90.00	3.10
	170	g	131	5.6	16.0	74.8	250.0	153.0	5.27
	6	oz							
non-fat milk, plain, vanilla	100	g	78	2.9	17.0	47.0	141.0	88.00	0.00
	227	g	177	6.7	38.7	107.0	320.0	200.0	0.00
	8	oz							
non-fat milk, fruit	100	g	83	5.1	15.0	72.0	234.0	140.0	0.17
	170	g	141	8.7	25.5	122.0	398.0	238.0	0.29
	6	oz							
Soy, yogurt, plain	100	g	94	3.5	16.0	35.0	47.00	38.00	1.80
	170	g	160	6.0	27.1	59.5	79.90	64.60	3.06
	6	oz							
Greek, plain, whole milk	100	g	97	9.0	4.0	35.0	141.0	135.0	5.00
	170	g	165	15.3	6.8	59.5	240.0	230.0	8.50
	6	oz							
Greek, fruit, whole milk	100	g	106	7.3	12.3	37.0	113.0	109.0	3.00
	170	g	180	12.5	20.9	62.9	192.0	185.0	5.10
	6	oz							
Greek, flavored, other than fruit	100	g	111	8.5	9.4	39.0	121.0	117.0	4.44
	170	g	189	14.4	15.9	66.3	206.0	199.0	7.55
	6	oz							
Greek, plain, low fat	100	g	73	10.0	3.9	34.0	141.0	137.0	1.92
	170	g	124	16.9	6.7	57.8	240.0	233.0	3.26
	6	oz							
Greek, LF, flavors other than fruit	100	g	95	8.6	9.5	40.0	123.0	119.0	2.50
	170	g	162	14.7	16.2	68.0	209.0	202.0	4.25
	6	oz							
Greek, non-fat (NF), plain	100	g	59	10.2	3.6	36.0	141.0	135.0	0.39
	170	g	100	17.3	6.1	61.2	240.0	230.0	0.66
	6	oz							
Greek, NF, flavors other than fruit	100	g	78	8.6	10.4	34.0	123.0	119.0	0.18
	170	g	133	14.7	17.6	57.8	209.0	202.0	0.31
	6	oz							
Frozen yogurt, chocolate	100	g	131	3.0	21.6	63.0	234.0	89.00	3.60
	160	g	210	4.8	34.6	101.0	374.0	142.0	5.76
1 scoop= small cup	1	scoop							

YOGURT

	SERVING QUANTITY	SERVING UNIT	CALORIES (kcal)	PROTEIN (g)	TOTAL CARBOHYDRATES (g)	SODIUM (mg)	POTASSIUM (mg)	PHOSPHORUS (mg)	TOTAL FAT (g)
Frozen yogurt, vanilla	100	g	127	3.0	21.6	63.0	156.0	89.00	3.60
	160	g	203	4.8	34.6	101.0	250.0	142.0	5.76
1 scoop= small cup	1	scoop							
Frozen yogurt, soft serve, chocolate	100	g	160	4.3	24.9	86.0	237.0	141.0	5.76
	175	g	280	7.5	43.5	150.0	415.0	247.0	10.10
	1	c							
Frozn yogurt, soft serve, vanilla	100	g	159	4.0	24.2	87.0	211.0	129.0	5.60
	175	g	278	7.0	42.4	152.0	369.0	226.0	9.80
	1	c							
Frozn yogurt bar, vanilla	100	g	127	3.0	21.6	63.0	156.0	89.00	3.60
	65	g	83	2.0	14.0	41.0	101.0	57.80	2.34
	1	bar							
Frozn yogurt bar, chocolate	100	g	131	3.0	21.6	63.0	234.0	89.00	3.60
	65	g	85	2.0	14.0	41.0	152.0	57.80	2.34
	1	bar							
Frozn yogurt cone, vanilla	100	g	139	3.2	23.9	71.0	154.0	89.00	3.73
	125	g	174	4.0	29.9	88.8	192.0	111.0	4.66
	1	cone							
Frozn yogurt cone, chocolate	100	g	142	3.2	23.9	71.0	229.0	89.00	3.73
	125	g	178	4.0	29.9	88.8	286.0	111.0	4.66
	1	cone							
Frozn yogurt, waffle cone, vanilla	100	g	143	3.3	25.3	77.0	155.0	90.00	3.61
	255	g	365	8.4	64.5	196.0	395.0	230.0	9.20
	1	cone							
Frozn yogurt, waffle cone, choco	100	g	147	3.3	25.3	77.0	229.0	90.00	3.61
	255	g	375	8.4	64.5	196.0	584.0	230.0	9.20
	1	cone							

YOGURT

	SERVING QUANTITY	SERVING UNIT	CALORIES (kCal)	PROTEIN (g)	TOTAL CARBOHYDRATES (g)	SODIUM (mg)	POTASSIUM (mg)	PHOSPHORUS (mg)	TOTAL FAT (g)
coconut milk, yogurt	100	g	64	0.3	8.0	21.0	27.00	2.00	3.50
	170	g	109	0.5	13.5	35.7	45.90	3.40	5.95
	6	oz							
dressing	100	g	220	3.5	11.8	43.0	146.0	85.00	18.27
	15.4	g	34	0.5	1.8	6.6	22.50	13.10	2.81
	1	tbsp							
liquid	100	g	72	3.7	11.8	53.0	171.0	103.0	1.09
	245	g	176	9.1	28.9	130.0	419.0	252.0	2.67
	1	c							
plain, whole milk	100	g	61	3.5	4.7	46.0	155.0	95.00	3.25
	227	g	138	7.9	10.6	104.0	352.0	216.0	7.38
	8	oz							
	100	g	87	3.1	12.4	44.0	146.0	86.00	2.87
Whole milk with fruit			14						
	170	g	8	5.3	21.0	74.8	248.0	146.0	4.88
	6	oz							

CHEESE

	SERVING QUANTITY	SERVING UNIT	CALORIES (kCal)	PROTEIN (g)	TOTAL CARBOHYDRATES (g)	SODIUM (mg)	POTASSIUM (mg)	PHOSPHORUS (mg)	TOTAL FAT (g)
Cheddar, reduced	100	g	398	24.4	1.9	21.0	112.00	484.0	32.62
sodium	21	g	84	5.1	0.4	4.4	23.50	102.0	6.85
	1	slice							
Cheddar, sharp	100	g	410	24.3	2.1	644.0	76.00	460.0	33.82
sliced	28	g	115	6.8	0.6	180.0	21.30	129.0	9.47
	1	oz							
Cheddar/	100	g	290	16.4	8.7	1625	242.00	875.0	21.23
American cheese	21	g	61	3.5	1.8	341.0	50.80	184.0	4.46
spread									
	1	wedge							
American	100	g	307	16.1	8.9	1279.	295.00	768.0	23.06
	21	g	65	3.4	1.9	269.0	62.00	161.0	4.84
	1	slice							
Brick	100	g	371	23.2	2.8	560.0	136.00	451.0	29.68
	17.2	g	64	4.0	0.5	96.3	23.40	77.60	5.10
	1	cubic inch							
Monterey	100	g	373	24.5	0.7	600.0	81.00	444.0	30.28
shredded	113	g	421	27.7	0.8	678.0	91.50	502.0	34.20
	1	cup							
Cheddar	100	g	408	23.3	2.4	654.0	77.00	458.0	34.00
	21	g	86	4.9	0.5	137.0	16.20	96.20	7.14
	1	slice							
Colby	100	g	394	23.8	2.6	604.0	127.00	457.0	32.11
	21	g	83	5.0	0.5	127.0	26.70	96.00	6.74
	1	slice							
Caraway	100	g	376	25.2	1.1	690.0	93.00	490.0	29.20
	28.35	g	107	7.1	0.9	196.0	26.40	139.0	8.28
	1	oz							
Edam	100	g	356	24.9	2.2	819.0	121.00	546.0	27.44
	21	g	75	5.2	0.5	172.0	25.40	115.0	5.76
	1	slice							
Fontina	100	g	389	25.6	1.6	800.0	64.00	346.0	31.14
	21	g	82	5.4	0.3	168.0	13.40	72.70	6.54
	1	slice							

CHEESE

	SERVING QUANTITY	SERVING UNIT	CALORIES (kcal)	PROTEIN (g)	TOTAL CARBOHYDRATES (g)	SODIUM (mg)	POTASSIUM (mg)	PHOSPHORUS (mg)	TOTAL FAT (g)
Gouda	100	g	356	24.9	2.2	819.0	121.0	546.0	27.44
	28.35	g	101	7.0	0.6	232.0	34.30	155.0	7.78
	1	oz							
Gruyere	100	g	413	29.8	0.4	714.0	81.00	605.0	32.34
	21	g	87	6.3	0.1	150.0	17.00	127.0	6.70
	1	slice							
Blue or Roquefort	100	g	353	21.4	2.3	1146.0	256.0	387.0	28.74
	17.3	g	61	3.7	0.4	198.0	44.30	67.00	4.97
	1	cubic inch							
Colby Jack	100	g	384	24.1	1.6	602.0	104.0	450.0	31.20
	21	g	81	5.1	0.3	126.0	21.80	94.50	6.55
	1	slice							
Parmesan, grated	100	g	420	29.6	12.4	1750.0	184.0	634.0	28.00
	7.6	g	32	2.3	0.9	133.0	14.00	48.20	1.82
	1	tbsp							
Parmesan, hard	100	g	421	29.6	12.4	1750.0	184.0	634.0	28.00
	10.3	g	43	3.1	1.3	180.0	19.00	65.30	2.88
	1	cubic inch							
Mexican blend shredded	100	g	358	23.5	1.8	607.0	85.00	438.0	28.51
	113	g	405	26.6	2.0	686.0	96.00	495.0	32.20
	1	cup							
Mexican blend, reduced fat shredded	100	g	282	24.7	3.4	776.0	93.00	583.0	19.40
	113	g	319	27.9	3.9	877.0	105.0	659.0	21.90
	1	cup							
Muenster	100	g	368	23.4	1.1	628.0	134.0	468.0	30.04
	21	g	77	5.0	0.2	132.0	28.10	98.30	6.31
	1	slice							
Provolone	100	g	351	25.6	2.1	727.0	138.0	496.0	26.62
	21	g	74	5.4	0.4	153.0	29.00	104.0	5.59
	1	slice							
Romano	100	g	387	31.8	3.6	1433.0	86.00	760.0	26.94
	28.35	g	110	9.0	1.0	406.0	24.40	215.0	7.64
	1	oz							
Swiss	100	g	393	27.0	1.4	185.0	71.00	574.0	31.00
	21	g	83	5.7	0.3	38.8	14.90	121.0	6.51
	1	slice							
Tilsiter/ Tilsit	100	g	340	24.4	1.9	753.0	65.00	500.0	25.98
	28.35	g	96	6.9	0.5	213.0	18.40	142.0	7.36
	1	oz							

COCONUT	SERVING QUANTITY	SERVING UNIT	CALORIES (KCal)	PROTEIN (g)	TOTAL CARBOHYDRATES (g)	SODIUM (mg)	POTASSIUM (mg)	PHOSPHORUS (mg)	TOTAL FAT (g)
fresh	100	g	354	3.3	15.2	20.00	356.0	113.0	33.5
	85	g	301	2.8	12.9	17.00	303.0	96.00	28.5
	1	c							
water, unsweetened	100	g	18	0.2	4.2	26.00	165.0	5.00	0.0
	240	g	43	0.5	10.2	62.40	396.0	12.00	0.0
	1	c							
milk	100	g	31	0.2	2.9	19.00	19.00	0.00	2.1
	244	g	76	0.5	7.1	46.40	46.40	0.00	5.1
	1	c							
milk/cream **for cooking**	100	g	230	2.3	5.5	15.00	263.0	100.0	23.8
	240	g	552	5.5	13.3	36.00	631.0	240.0	57.2
	1	c							
yogurt	100	g	64	0.3	8.0	21.00	27.00	2.00	3.5
	170	g	109	0.5	13.5	35.70	45.90	3.40	6.0
	6	oz							
cream, canned, sweetened	100	g	357	1.2	53.2	36.00	101.0	22.00	16.3
	37	g	132	0.4	19.7	13.30	37.40	8.14	6.0
	1/4	c							
oil	100	g	833	0.0	0.0	0.00	0.00	0.00	99.1
	14	g	117	0.0	0.0	0.00	0.00	0.00	13.9
	1	tbsp							
flaked, shredded, packed	100	g	456	3.1	51.9	285.0	361.0	100.0	28.0
	28	g	128	1.0	14.5	79.80	101.0	28.00	7.8
	2	tbsp							

F. FATS and OILS

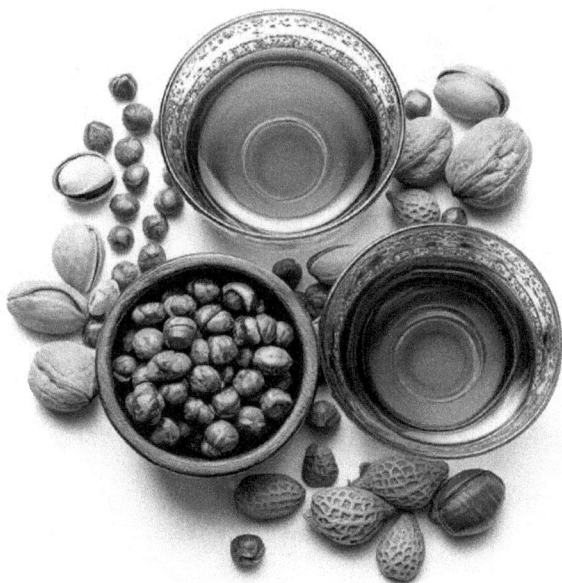

ALMOND	SERVING QUANTITY	SERVING UNIT	CALORIES (kCal)	PROTEIN (g)	TOTAL CARBOHYDRATES (g)	SODIUM (mg)	POTASSIUM (mg)	PHOSPHORUS (mg)	TOTAL FAT (g)
whole	100	g	579	21.2	21.6	1.00	733.00	481.00	49.9
	35.75	g	207	7.6	7.7	0.36	262.05	171.96	17.9
	0.25	c							
slivered	100	g	579	21.2	21.6	1.00	733.00	481.00	49.9
	27	g	156	5.7	5.8	0.27	197.91	129.87	13.5
	0.25	c							
ground	100	g	579	21.2	21.6	1.00	733.00	481.00	49.9
	23.75	g	138	5.0	5.1	0.24	174.09	114.42	11.9
	0.25	c							
paste (marzipan)	100	g	458	9.0	47.8	9.00	314.00	258.00	27.7
	28.38	g	130	2.6	13.6	2.55	89.10	73.21	7.9
	2	tbsp							
oil	100	g	884	0.0	0.0	0.00	0.00	0.00	100.0
	13.6	g	120	0.0	0.0	0.00	0.00	0.00	13.6
	1	tbsp							
butter, without salt added	100	g	614	21.0	18.8	227.0	748.00	508.00	55.5
	16	g	98	3.4	3.0	1.12	119.68	81.28	8.9
	1	tbsp							
dry roasted, without salt added	100	g	598	3.0	21.0	3.00	713.00	471.00	52.5
	34.5	g	206	7.2	7.3	1.04	245.99	162.50	18.1
	0.25	c							
oil roasted, without salt	100	g	607	21.2	17.7	1.00	699.00	466.00	55.2
	39.25	g	238	8.3	6.9	0.39	274.36	182.91	21.7
	0.25	c							
milk, unsweetened, shelf stable	100	g	15	0.4	1.3	72.00	67.00	9.00	1.0
	262	g	39	1.1	3.4	188.6	175.54	23.58	2.5
	1	c							
milk, sweetened, vanilla flavor ready-to-drink	100	g	38	0.4	6.6	63.00	50.00	8.00	1.0
	240	g	91	1.0	15.8	151.2	120.00	19.20	2.5
	1	c							
milk, chocolate flavor, unsweetened fortified Vit. D2 and E	100	g	21	0.8	1.3	75.00	96.00	17.00	1.5
	240	g	50	2.0	3.0	180.0	130.40	40.80	3.5
	1	c							

WALNUT	SERVING QUANTITY	SERVING UNIT	CALORIES (kCal)	PROTEIN (g)	TOTAL CARBOHYDRATES (g)	SODIUM (mg)	POTASSIUM (mg)	PHOSPHORUS (mg)	TOTAL FAT (g)
english, halves	100	g	654	15.2	13.7	2.00	441.00	346.0	65.2
	25	g	164	3.8	3.4	0.50	110.25	86.50	16.3
	0.25	c							
english, ground	100	g	654	15.2	13.7	2.00	441.00	346.0	65.2
	20	g	131	3.1	2.7	0.40	88.20	69.20	13.0
	0.25	c							
english, chopped	100	g	654	15.2	13.7	2.00	441.00	346.0	65.2
	29.25	g	191	4.5	4.0	0.59	128.99	101.2	19.1
	0.25	c							
butternut or white walnut, dried	100	g	612	24.9	12.1	1.00	421.00	446.0	57.0
	120	g	734	29.9	14.5	1.20	505.20	535.2	68.4
	1	c							
black or american, dried, chopped	100	g	619	24.1	9.6	2.00	523.00	513.0	59.3
	31.25	g	193	7.5	3.0	0.63	163.44	160.3	18.5
	0.25	c							
black or american, dried, ground	100	g	604	23.5	9.3	1.95	509.92	500.2	57.9
	26.67	g	161	6.3	2.5	0.52	135.98	133.4	15.4
	0.33	c							
glazed	100	g	500	8.3	47.6	446.0	232.00	na	35.7
	28.35	g	142	2.4	13.5	126.5	65.77	na	10.1
	1	oz							
oil	100	g	884	0.0	0.0	0.0	0.00	0.00	100.0
	13.6	g	120	0.0	0.0	0.0	0.00	0.00	13.6
	1	tbsp							
CHIA									
seeds, dried	100	g	486	16.5	42.1	16.00	407.00	860.0	30.7
	28.35	g	138	4.7	11.9	4.54	115.38	243.8	8.7
	1	oz							

OLIVE	SERVING QUANTITY	SERVING UNIT	CALORIES (kCal)	PROTEIN (g)	TOTAL CARBOHYDRATES (g)	SODIUM (mg)	POTASSIUM (mg)	PHOSPHORUS (mg)	TOTAL FAT (g)
oil, extra virgin,	100	g	884	0.0	0.0	2.00	1.00	0.00	100.0
virgin	14	g	124	0.0	0.0	0.28	0.14	0.00	14.0
	1	tbsp							
black, kalamata	100	g	116	0.8	6.0	735.0	8.00	3.00	10.9
	15	g	17	0.1	0.9	110.0	1.20	0.45	1.6
	3	pcs							
green	100	g	145	1.0	3.8	1556	42.00	4.00	15.3
	15	g	22	0.2	0.6	233	6.30	0.60	2.3
	3	pcs							
spread	100	g	278	0.7	4.2	835	17.00	3.00	30.1
(tapenade)	16	g	45	0.1	0.7	134	2.72	0.48	4.8
	1	tbsp							
stuffed	100	g	128	1.0	4.0	1340	58.00	6.00	13.2
	15	g	19	0.2	0.6	201	8.70	0.90	2.0
	3	pcs							

COCONUT

	SERVING QUANTITY	SERVING UNIT	CALORIES (kCal)	PROTEIN (g)	TOTAL CARBOHYDRATES (g)	SODIUM (mg)	POTASSIUM (mg)	PHOSPHORUS (mg)	TOTAL FAT (g)
fresh	100	g	354	3.3	15.2	20.00	356.0	113.0	33.5
	85	g	301	2.8	12.9	17.00	303.0	96.00	28.5
	1	c							
water,	100	g	18	0.2	4.2	26.00	165.0	5.00	0.0
unsweetened	240	g	43	0.5	10.2	62.40	396.0	12.00	0.0
	1	c							
milk	100	g	31	0.2	2.9	19.00	19.00	0.00	2.1
	244	g	76	0.5	7.1	46.40	46.40	0.00	5.1
	1	c							
milk/cream for	100	g	230	2.3	5.5	15.00	263.0	100.0	23.8
cooking	240	g	552	5.5	13.3	36.00	631.0	240.0	57.2
	1	c							
yogurt	100	g	64	0.3	8.0	21.00	27.00	2.00	3.5
	170	g	109	0.5	13.5	35.70	45.90	3.40	6.0
	6	oz							
cream, canned,	100	g	357	1.2	53.2	36.00	101.0	22.00	16.3
sweetened	37	g	132	0.4	19.7	13.30	37.40	8.14	6.0
	1/4	c							
oil	100	g	833	0.0	0.0	0.00	0.00	0.00	99.1
	14	g	117	0.0	0.0	0.00	0.00	0.00	13.9
	1	tbsp							
flaked,	100	g	456	3.1	51.9	285.00	361.0	100.0	28.0
shredded, packed	28	g	128	1.0	14.5	79.80	101.0	28.00	7.8
	2	tbsp							

PECANS	SERVING QUANTITY	SERVING UNIT	CALORIES (kcal)	PROTEIN (g)	TOTAL CARBOHYDRATES (g)	SODIUM (mg)	POTASSIUM (mg)	PHOSPHORUS (mg)	TOTAL FAT (g)
chopped	100	g	691	9.2	13.9	0.00	410.0	277.0	72.0
	109	g	753	10.0	15.1	0.00	446.9	410.0	78.5
	1	c							
halves	100	g	691	9.2	13.9	0.00	410.0	277.0	72.0
	24.75	g	171	2.3	3.4	0.00	101.5	68.56	17.8
	0.25	c							
halves, oil roasted	100	g	715	9.2	13.0	1.00	392.0	263.0	75.2
	110	g	787	10.1	14.3	1.10	431.2	289.3	82.8
	1	c							
dry roasted, without salt added	100	g	710	9.5	13.6	1.00	424.0	293.0	74.3
	28.35	g	201	2.7	3.8	0.28	120.2	83.07	21.1
	1	oz							
MACADAMIA									
whole or halves (1 oz = 10-12 kernels)	100	g	718	7.9	13.8	5.00	368.0	188.0	75.8
	134	g	962	10.6	18.5	6.70	493.1	251.9	101.5
	1	c							
dry roasted, without salt added	100	g	718	7.8	13.4	4.00	363.0	198.0	76.1
	33.5	g	241	2.6	4.5	1.34	121.6	66.33	25.5
	0.25	c							
FLAXSEED									
seeds, whole	100	g	534	18.3	28.9	30.00	813.0	642.0	42.2
	10.3	g	55	1.9	3.0	3.09	83.70	66.10	4.3
	1	tbsp							
seeds, ground	7	g	37	1.3	2.0	2.10	56.90	44.90	3.0
	1	tbsp							
oil	100	g	884	0.1	0.0	0.00	0.00	1.00	100.0
	14	g	124	0.0	0.0	0.00	0.00	0.14	14.0
	1	tbsp							
oil with added sliced flaxseed	100	g	878	0.4	0.4	6.00	31.00	27.00	99.0
	13.7	g	120	0.1	0.1	0.82	4.25	3.70	13.6
	1	tbsp							
oil, cold pressed	100	g	884	0.1	0.0	0.00	0.00	1.00	100.0
	13.6	g	120	0.0	0.0	0.00	0.00	0.14	13.6
	1	tbsp							

PUMPKIN	SERVING QUANTITY	SERVING UNIT	CALORIES (kcal)	PROTEIN (g)	TOTAL CARBOHYDRATES (g)	SODIUM (mg)	POTASSIUM (mg)	PHOSPHORUS (mg)	TOTAL FAT (g)
meat, 1" cubes	100	g	26	1.0	6.5	1.00	340.0	44.00	0.1
	116	g	30	1.2	7.5	1.16	394.4	51.04	0.1
	1	c							
flowers	100	g	15	1.0	3.3	5.00	173.0	49.00	0.1
	33	g	1	0.0	0.1	0.20	6.92	1.96	0.0
	1	c							
meat, boiled, drained, no salt added	100	g	20	0.7	4.9	1.00	230.0	30.00	0.1
	122.5	g	25	0.9	6.0	1.23	281.7	36.75	0.1
	0.5	c							
pumpkin pie spice powder	100	g	342	5.8	69.3	52.00	663.0	118.0	12.6
	1.7	g	6	0.1	1.2	0.88	11.27	2.01	0.2
	1	tsp							
seed sunfish, cooked dry heat	100	g	114	24.9	0.0	103.0	449.0	231.00	0.9
	85.05	g	97	21.2	0.0	87.60	381.8	196.46	0.8
	3	oz							
seeds, kernels, whole, roasted without salt added	100	g	446	18.6	53.8	18.00	919.0	92.00	19.4
	32	g	143	5.9	17.2	5.76	294.0	29.44	6.2
	0.5	c							

AVOCADO

	SERVING QUANTITY	SERVING UNIT	CALORIES (kCal)	PROTEIN (g)	TOTAL CARBOHYDRATES (g)	SODIUM (mg)	POTASSIUM (mg)	PHOSPHORUS (mg)	TOTAL FAT (g)
fresh, raw	100.0	g	160	2.0	8.5	7.00	485.0	52.00	14.66
mashed/ pureed	230.0	g	368	4.6	19.6	16.1	1,120.0	120.0	33.70
	1.00	c							
oil	100.0	g	884	0.0	0.0	0.00	0.00	0.00	100.00
	14.00	g	124	0.0	0.0	0.00	0.00	0.00	14.00
	1.00	tbsp							
dressing	100.0	g	427	1.9	7.4	867	58.00	31.00	43.33
	15.30	g	65	0.3	1.1	133.	8.87	4.74	6.63
	1.00	tbsp							
California, raw/fresh no seed and skin	100.0	g	167	2.0	8.6	8.00	507.0	54.00	15.41
	136.0	g	227	2.7	11.8	10.9	690.0	73.40	21.00
	1.00	pc/ item							
Florida, fresh/ raw no seed and skin	100.0	g	120	2.2	7.8	2.00	351.0	40.00	10.06
	304.0	g	365	6.8	23.8	6.08	1,070.0	122.0	30.60
	1.00	pc/ item							
Guacamole	100.0	g	155	2.0	8.5	344	472.0	51.00	14.18
	15.00	g	23	0.3	1.3	51.6	70.80	7.65	2.13
	1.00	tbsp							

G. HERBS and SPICES

	SERVING QUANTITY	SERVING UNIT	CALORIES (kCal)	PROTEIN (g)	TOTAL CARBOHYDRATES (g)	SODIUM (mg)	POTASSIUM (mg)	PHOSPHORUS (mg)	TOTAL FAT (g)
SAGE									
ground	100	g	315	10.6	60.7	11	1070	91	12.8
1 Tbsp	2	g	6.3	0.21	1.21	0.22	21.4	1.82	0.256
CINNAMON									
ground	100	g	247	3.99	80.6	10	431	64	1.24
1 Tbsp	7.8	g	19.3	0.31	6.29	0.78	33.6	4.99	0.097
CUMIN									
seed	100	g	375	17.8	44.2	168	1790	499	22.3
1 Tbsp Whole	6	g	22.5	1.07	2.65	10.1	107	29.9	1.34
NUTMEG									
ground	100	g	525	5.84	49.3	16	350	213	36.3
1 tsp	7	g	36.8	0.41	3.45	1.12	24.5	14.9	2.54
CLOVES									
ground	100	g	274	5.97	65.5	277	1020	104	13
1tsp	6.5	g	17.8	0.39	4.26	18	66.3	6.76	0.845
PARSLEY									
fresh	100	g	36	2.97	6.33	56	554	58	0.79
dried	100	g	292	26.6	50.6	452	2680	436	5.48
CORIANDER									
seed	100	g	298	12.4	55	35	1270	409	17.8
leaves, raw	100	g	23	2.13	3.67	46	521	48	0.52
THYME									
fresh	100	g	101	5.56	24.4	9	609	106	1.68
dried	100	g	276	9.11	63.9	55	814	201	7.43
LEMON GRASS									
citronella, raw	100	g	99	1.82	25.3	6	723	101	0.49

	SERVING QUANTITY	SERVING UNIT	CALORIES (kcal)	PROTEIN (g)	TOTAL CARBOHYDRATES (g)	SODIUM (mg)	POTASSIUM (mg)	PHOSPHORUS (mg)	TOTAL FAT (g)
ONION									
red, raw	100	g	44	0.94	9.93	1	197	41	0.1
1 onion	197	g	86.7	1.85	19.6	1.97	388	80.8	0.197
white, raw	100	g	36	0.89	7.68	2	141	29	0.13
yellow, raw	100	g	38	0.83	8.61	1	182	34	0.05
1 onion	143	g	54.3	1.19	12.3	1.43	260	48.6	0.071
GARLIC									
raw	100	g	149	6.36	33.1	17	401	153	0.5
3 cloves	9	g	13.4	0.572	2.98	1.53	36.1	13.8	0.045
GINGER									
raw	100	g	80	1.82	17.8	13	415	34	0.75
SPRING ONIONS									
raw	100	g	32	1.83	7.34	16	276	37	0.19
1 large	25	g	8	0.458	1.84	4	69	9.25	0.048
CHIVES									
raw	100	g	30	3.27	4.35	3	296	58	0.73
BASIL									
fresh	100	g	23	3.15	2.65	4	295	56	0.64
dried	100	g	233	23	47.8	76	2630	274	4.07
OREGANO									
dried	100	g	265	9	68.9	25	1260	148	4.28
ROSEMARY									
fresh	100	g	131	3.31	20.7	26	668	66	5.86
dried	100	g	331	4.88	64.1	50	995	70	15.2
MARJORAM									
dried	100	g	271	12.7	60.6	77	1520	306	7.04

	SERVING QUANTITY	SERVING UNIT	CALORIES (kCal)	PROTEIN (g)	TOTAL CARBOHYDRATES (g)	SODIUM (mg)	POTASSIUM (mg)	PHOSPHORUS (mg)	TOTAL FAT (g)
FENNEL									
Bulb, raw	100	g	31	1.24	7.3	52	414	50	0.2
seed	100	g	345	15.8	52.3	88	1690	487	14.9
1 Tbsp	5.8	g	20	0.92	3.03	5.1	98	28	0.864
DILL									
weed, fresh	100	g	43	3.46	7.02	61	738	66	1.12
weed, dried	100	g	253	20	55.8	208	3310	543	4.36
1 Tbsp	3.1	g	7.8	0.62	1.73	6.45	103	16.8	0.135
ANISE									
seed	100	g	337	17.6	50	16	1440	440	15.9
1 Tbsp	6.7	g	22.6	1.18	3.35	1.07	96.5	29.5	1.06
CARDAMOM									
spices	100	g	311	10.8	68.5	18	1120	229	6.7
1 Tbsp	5.8	g	18	0.63	3.97	1.04	65	10.3	0.389
CAYENNE									
pepper, red or cayenne	100	g	318	12	56.6	30	2010	293	17.3
1 tbsp	5.3	g	16.9	0.64	3	1.59	107	15.5	0.917
CURRY POWDER									
	100	g	325	14.3	55.8	52	1170	367	14
1 tbsp	6.3	g	20.5	0.90	3.52	3.28	73.7	23.1	0.882
PAPRIKA									
ground	100	g	282	14.1	54	68	2280	314	12.9
1 tbsp	6.8	g	19.2	0.96	3.67	4.62	155	21.4	0.877
CELERY									
celery, raw	100	g	14	0.69	2.97	80	260	24	0.17

	SERVING QUANTITY	SERVING UNIT	CALORIES (kCal)	PROTEIN (g)	TOTAL CARBOHYDRATES (g)	SODIUM (mg)	POTASSIUM (mg)	PHOSPHORUS (mg)	TOTAL FAT (g)
SAFFRON									
	100	g	310	11.4	65.4	148	1720	252	5.85
1 tbsp	2.1	g	6.51	0.24	1.37	3.11	36.1	5.29	0.123
PEPPER, BLACK									
ground	100	g	251	10.4	64	20	1330	158	3.26
1 tbsp	6.9	g	17.3	0.72	4.42	1.38	91.8	10.9	0.225
PEPPER, WHITE									
ground	100	g	296	10.4	68.6	5	73	176	2.12
1 tbsp	7.1	g	21	0.74	4.87	0.355	5.18	12.5	0.151
TARRAGON									
dried	100	g	295	22.8	50.2	62	3020	313	7.24
1 Tbsp, leaves	1.8	g	5.31	0.41	0.904	1.12	54.4	5.63	0.13
1 Tbsp, ground	4.8	g	14.2	1.09	2.41	2.98	145	15	0.348
HORSERADISH									
	100	g	48	1.18	11.3	420	246	31	0.69
1 tbsp	15	g	7.2	0.18	1.7	63	36.9	4.65	0.103

Complete List of High Lectin Foods to Avoid

These foods are high in lectins and should be limited or avoided by those following a low lectin diet:

Fruits

Bananas (unripe)

Blackberries

Figs

Elderberries

Avocados (ripe)

Vegetables

Tomatoes

Potatoes (white and red)

Eggplants

Peas

Peppers (hot varieties)

Sweet potatoes

Legumes

Beans (all types, including kidney, black, and navy beans)

Lentils

Peas

Soybeans (and soy products)

Grains

Whole wheat products

Barley

Rye

Quinoa (in large quantities)

Bulgur

Nuts and Seeds

Peanuts

Cashews

Sunflower seeds

Understanding the differences between low and high lectin foods can empower you to make informed dietary choices. By focusing on low-lectin options and being mindful of the impact of lectins on your health, you can optimize your nutrition and improve your well-being.

Chapter 5: Meal Planning Made Easy

The Importance of Meal Planning

Statistics show that **up to 70% of individuals** who adopt a new dietary regimen find meal planning to be a crucial factor in their success. For those following a low lectin diet, effective meal planning can significantly enhance adherence to dietary guidelines and improve overall health outcomes. By taking the time to plan meals, individuals can make informed choices about their food intake, avoid high-lectin foods, and ensure they are consuming a balanced variety of nutrients.

Introduction to Meal Planning

Meal planning is an essential tool for anyone looking to maintain a specific diet, particularly one that eliminates or reduces certain food components like lectins. A well-structured meal plan not only simplifies grocery shopping but also reduces the stress of daily cooking. By planning ahead, you can ensure that you have all the necessary ingredients on hand, minimizing the temptation to resort to high-lectin convenience foods.

Here are some benefits of meal planning:

Saves Time: With a plan in place, you can prepare multiple meals at once, reducing cooking time during the week.

Reduces Food Waste: Planning helps you use ingredients efficiently, decreasing the likelihood of spoilage and waste.

Encourages Healthy Choices: When you plan your meals, you are more likely to choose low lectin foods and maintain a balanced diet.

How to Create Your Own Low Lectin Meal Plans

Creating your own low lectin meal plan can be a straightforward process. Here's a step-by-step guide to help you get started:

1. **Assess Your Dietary Needs**: Consider any specific health goals, dietary restrictions, or preferences. This will guide your food choices and meal planning.

2. **Choose Low Lectin Foods**: Refer to the low lectin food list from Chapter 4. Select a variety of foods from different categories, including fruits, vegetables, proteins, and grains.

3. **Plan for the Week**:

   Breakfast: Consider options like smoothies with low lectin fruits or eggs with sautéed vegetables.

   Lunch: Think about salads with grilled chicken or quinoa bowls with roasted vegetables.

   Dinner: Plan meals like baked salmon with asparagus or stir-fried tofu with bell peppers.

   Snacks: Include low lectin snacks like rice cakes with nut butter or vegetable sticks with hummus.

4. **Create a Grocery List**: Once your meals are planned, make a shopping list of the ingredients you will need. This will help you stay organized and ensure you have everything on hand.

5. **Prepare in Advance**: If possible, prepare some meals or ingredients in advance. For example, you can chop vegetables, cook grains, or batch-cook proteins to make meal assembly quicker during the week.

6. **Stay Flexible**: Life can be unpredictable, so be open to adjusting your meal plan as needed. If you have leftovers, incorporate them into your next meals to reduce waste.

Tips for Cooking with Low Lectin Ingredients

Cooking with low lectin ingredients can be both enjoyable and rewarding. Here are some tips to help you create delicious meals while adhering to your dietary restrictions:

1. **Use Fresh Ingredients**: Fresh fruits and vegetables are typically lower in lectins and higher in nutrients. Aim to incorporate a variety of colors and types into your meals.

2. **Experiment with Herbs and Spices**: Enhance the flavor of your dishes with fresh herbs and low-lectin spices. Options like basil, oregano, garlic, and ginger can elevate your meals without adding lectins.

3. **Focus on Cooking Methods**: Opt for cooking methods that preserve the nutritional value of low lectin foods. Steaming, grilling, roasting, and sautéing are excellent choices.

4. **Balance Your Plate**: Aim for a balanced plate that includes a source of protein, healthy fats, and a variety of low lectin vegetables. This not only ensures nutritional adequacy but also makes meals more satisfying.

5. **Portion Size Matters**: Be mindful of serving sizes, as even low lectin foods can contribute to overall lectin intake if consumed in large quantities.

6. **Get Creative**: Don't hesitate to try new recipes and cooking techniques. Look for inspiration in cookbooks, blogs, and social media focused on low lectin eating.

By implementing these meal planning strategies and cooking tips, you can enjoy a varied and delicious low lectin diet that supports your health and well-being.

Chapter 6: 7-Day Meal Plan

As more individuals recognize the impact of diet on health, the low lectin lifestyle has gained traction, particularly among those seeking to alleviate digestive issues and reduce inflammation. Studies show that **over 40% of adults** actively seek dietary changes to improve their health and well-being, with many turning to low lectin foods as part of their journey.

Imagine Sarah, a busy professional in her 50s, who struggled with bloating and fatigue. After embracing a low lectin diet, she found that meal planning was the key to her success. By dedicating time to organize her meals, she not only simplified her grocery shopping but also discovered new flavors and recipes that nourished her body and energized her days.

In this chapter, you will find a comprehensive **7-Day Meal Plan** designed to help you seamlessly incorporate low lectin foods into your routine. Each day features balanced meals and snacks that promote health while ensuring variety and satisfaction. Let's embark on this flavorful journey together and make healthy eating an enjoyable part of your lifestyle!

Sample Meal Plan for One Week

Day 1	
Breakfast: Greek yogurt with blueberries and a sprinkle of cinnamon **Snack:** Apple slices with almond butter **Lunch:** Grilled chicken salad with mixed greens, cucumber, and olive oil dressing **Snack:** Rice cakes with cream cheese **Dinner:** Baked salmon with roasted zucchini and quinoa	Daily Totals: Calories: 1,700 Protein: 100g Fat: 70g Carbohydrates: 170g Fiber: 25g Sodium: 900mg Potassium: 3,200mg

Day 2	
Breakfast: Smoothie with spinach, banana, almond milk, and almond butter **Snack:** Celery sticks with hummus **Lunch:** Quinoa bowl with grilled shrimp, bell peppers, and avocado **Snack:** Handful of walnuts **Dinner:** Stir-fried tofu with broccoli and cauliflower rice	*Daily Totals:* Calories: 1,600 Protein: 80g Fat: 65g Carbohydrates: 150g Fiber: 30g Sodium: 800mg Potassium: 3,000mg

Day 3	
Breakfast: Oatmeal made with almond milk, topped with sliced bananas **Snack:** Cucumber slices with guacamole **Lunch:** Turkey lettuce wraps with avocado, tomato, and mustard **Snack:** Hard-boiled eggs **Dinner:** Grilled chicken thighs with roasted carrots and steamed asparagus	*Daily Totals:* Calories: 1,650 Protein: 90g Fat: 60g Carbohydrates: 160g Fiber: 28g Sodium: 700mg Potassium: 3,200mg

Day 4	
Breakfast: Scrambled eggs with sautéed spinach and mushrooms **Snack:** Mixed berries (strawberries, blueberries, raspberries) **Lunch:** Zucchini noodles with marinara sauce and grilled chicken **Snack:** Rice cakes topped with almond butter **Dinner:** Baked cod with lemon and herbs, served with quinoa and green beans	*Daily Totals:* Calories: 1,600 Protein: 85g Fat: 55g Carbohydrates: 140g Fiber: 26g Sodium: 750mg Potassium: 3,400mg

Day 5	
Breakfast: Chia seed pudding made with almond milk, topped with kiwi **Snack:** Bell pepper slices with hummus **Lunch:** Grilled salmon salad with mixed greens, avocado, and olive oil **Snack:** Handful of almonds **Dinner:** Stuffed bell peppers with ground turkey, rice, and spices	*Daily Totals:* Calories: 1,700 Protein: 95g Fat: 65g Carbohydrates: 150g Fiber: 30g Sodium: 850mg Potassium: 3,500mg

Day 6	
Breakfast: Smoothie with kale, banana, and almond milk **Snack:** Sliced apples with almond butter **Lunch:** Quinoa salad with chickpeas, cucumber, and lemon dressing **Snack:** Hard-boiled eggs **Dinner:** Grilled chicken with roasted Brussels sprouts and sweet potato	*Daily Totals:* Calories: 1,650 Protein: 85g Fat: 60g Carbohydrates: 140g Fiber: 27g Sodium: 800mg Potassium: 3,300mg

Day 7	
Breakfast: Coconut yogurt with sliced strawberries and chia seeds **Snack:** Carrot sticks with hummus **Lunch:** Turkey and avocado salad with mixed greens and olive oil dressing **Snack:** Rice cakes topped with cream cheese **Dinner:** Cauliflower rice stir-fry with assorted vegetables and chicken	*Daily Totals:* Calories: 1,600 Protein: 90g Fat: 55g Carbohydrates: 140g Fiber: 28g Sodium: 700mg Potassium: 3,400mg

Summary of Weekly Totals

Total Calories: 11,650

Total Protein: 525g

Total Fat: 390g

Total Carbohydrates: 1,050g

Total Fiber: 194g

Average Sodium: 780mg

Average Potassium: 3,400mg

This 7-Day Low Lectin Meal Plan is designed to provide a balanced and nutritious approach to eating while minimizing lectin intake. Each day includes a variety of foods to ensure you receive essential nutrients and maintain a satisfying diet.

Chapter 7: 20 Delicious Low Lectin Recipes

Welcome to a culinary adventure that celebrates the vibrant flavors and nourishing qualities of low lectin foods! In this chapter, we invite you to explore 20 delicious low lectin recipes that are not only easy to prepare but also designed to tantalize your taste buds while supporting your health. Whether you are new to the low lectin diet or a seasoned enthusiast, these recipes will inspire you to create meals that are both satisfying and healthful.

Eating well doesn't have to be a compromise. With the right ingredients and creative recipes, you can enjoy a wide variety of dishes that promote wellness without sacrificing flavor. From hearty breakfasts that kickstart your day to satisfying dinners that bring the family together, this collection covers all your meal needs.

Each recipe is crafted with care, focusing on wholesome ingredients that are low in lectins but high in nutrition. You'll find fresh vegetables, lean proteins, and aromatic herbs that come together in delightful combinations. Whether you're preparing a quick snack or a festive family meal, these recipes will help you embrace a lifestyle that prioritizes your health and well-being.

So grab your apron and let's get cooking! Dive into these delicious recipes and discover how easy and enjoyable it can be to eat in a way that supports your health. Your journey to flavorful, low lectin cooking starts here!

Chia Seed Pudding with Coconut Milk and Berries

Ingredients

- 1/4 cup chia seeds
- 1 cup coconut milk (canned or carton; ensure it's unsweetened)
- 1 tablespoon honey or maple syrup (optional, adjust sweetness to taste)
- 1/2 teaspoon vanilla extract (optional)
- 1/2 cup mixed berries (such as blueberries, strawberries, or raspberries)
- Pinch of salt

Instructions

1. Mix the Ingredients: In a medium bowl or jar, combine the chia seeds, coconut milk, honey (if using), vanilla extract, and a pinch of salt. Stir well to ensure the chia seeds are evenly distributed.
2. Refrigerate: Cover the bowl or jar and refrigerate for at least 4 hours, or overnight. The chia seeds will absorb the liquid and create a thick, pudding-like texture.
3. Serve: Once the pudding has set, give it a good stir. Top with mixed berries just before serving. Enjoy!

1 serving (approximately 1 cup)

Nutritional Information (Approximate per serving)

- Calories: 280

- Protein: 5g

- Fat: 18g

- Carbohydrates: 28g

- Fiber: 10g

- Sugar: 6g (from honey and berries)

- Sodium: 35mg (varies based on coconut milk)

- Potassium: 400mg (11% DV)

- Phosphorus: 150mg (12% DV)

Why This Recipe is Good for Low-Lectin Dieters

Chia Seed Pudding with Coconut Milk and Berries is an excellent choice for those following a low-lectin diet. Chia seeds are low in lectins and high in fiber and omega-3 fatty acids, promoting digestive health and reducing inflammation. Coconut milk adds a creamy texture without introducing high-lectin ingredients, while the berries provide antioxidants and essential vitamins. This recipe is not only delicious but also nutrient-dense, making it a satisfying breakfast or snack option.

Scrambled Eggs with Spinach and Feta

Ingredients

- 2 large eggs
- 1 cup fresh spinach, chopped
- 1/4 cup feta cheese, crumbled
- 1 tablespoon olive oil or butter
- Salt and pepper, to taste
- 1/4 teaspoon garlic powder (optional)

Instructions

1. Sauté the Spinach: In a skillet, heat the olive oil or butter over medium heat. Add the chopped spinach and sauté for about 1-2 minutes until wilted. If using garlic powder, add it in during this step for extra flavor.
2. Beat the Eggs: In a bowl, whisk together the eggs, salt, and pepper until well combined.
3. Cook the Eggs: Pour the beaten eggs into the skillet with the sautéed spinach. Cook for about 2-3 minutes, stirring gently, until the eggs are just set but still creamy.
4. Add Feta: Sprinkle the crumbled feta cheese over the eggs and gently fold it in until just melted.
5. Serve: Remove from heat and serve immediately. Enjoy your delicious scrambled eggs!

1 serving (approximately 1 cup)

Nutritional Information (Approximate per serving)

- Calories: 250
- Protein: 16g
- Fat: 20g
- Carbohydrates: 3g
- Fiber: 1g
- Sugar: 1g
- Sodium: 400mg (varies based on added salt and feta)
- Potassium: 350mg (10% DV)
- Phosphorus: 250mg (20% DV)

Why This Recipe is Good for Low-Lectin Dieters

Scrambled Eggs with Spinach and Feta is a fantastic option for those following a low-lectin diet. Eggs are a great source of protein without lectins, while spinach is low in lectins and high in vitamins A, C, and K, along with important minerals. Feta cheese adds flavor and creaminess while being low in lactose, making it easier to digest for some individuals. This dish is not only quick and easy to prepare but also nutrient-dense, making it perfect for breakfast or a light meal.

Smoothie Bowl with Kale, Banana, and Almond Milk

Ingredients

- 1 cup fresh kale leaves, stems removed
- 1 ripe banana
- 1 cup unsweetened almond milk (or any low-lectin milk alternative)
- 1 tablespoon almond butter (optional, for added creaminess and flavor)
- 1 tablespoon chia seeds (optional, for added fiber and omega-3s)

Toppings (optional):
- Sliced fresh fruit (e.g., strawberries, blueberries)
- Granola (low-lectin variety)
- Nuts or seeds (e.g., sliced almonds, pumpkin seeds)
- Coconut flakes

Instructions

1. Blend the Ingredients: In a blender, combine the kale, banana, almond milk, almond butter (if using), and chia seeds (if using). Blend until smooth and creamy.
2. Adjust Consistency: If the mixture is too thick, add a little more almond milk until you reach your desired consistency.
3. Serve: Pour the smoothie into a bowl and add your desired toppings. Arrange the sliced fruit, granola, nuts, or coconut flakes artistically on top.
4. Enjoy: Grab a spoon and enjoy your nutritious smoothie bowl!

1 serving (approximately 1 bowl)

Nutritional Information (Approximate per serving)

- Calories: 300

- Protein: 7g

- Fat: 15g

- Carbohydrates: 40g

- Fiber: 9g

- Sugar: 15g (from banana and toppings)

- Sodium: 100mg (varies based on added salt and almond milk)

- Potassium: 600mg (17% DV)

- Phosphorus: 200mg (15% DV)

Why This Recipe is Good for Low-Lectin Dieters

The Smoothie Bowl with Kale, Banana, and Almond Milk is an excellent choice for those on a low-lectin diet. Kale is a nutrient-dense leafy green that is low in lectins and high in vitamins A, C, and K, as well as antioxidants. Bananas provide natural sweetness and potassium, contributing to heart health and muscle function. Almond milk and almond butter add creaminess and healthy fats without introducing high-lectin ingredients. This recipe is not only refreshing and satisfying but also a great way to incorporate greens into your diet while adhering to low-lectin principles.

Grilled Chicken Salad with Avocado and Mixed Greens

Ingredients

- 1 pound boneless, skinless chicken breasts
- 2 tablespoons olive oil
- Salt and pepper, to taste
- 1 teaspoon garlic powder (optional)
- 6 cups mixed greens (such as spinach, arugula, and romaine)
- 1 ripe avocado, diced
- 1 cup cherry tomatoes, halved
- 1/2 cucumber, sliced
- 1/4 red onion, thinly sliced (optional)
- Juice of 1 lemon (for dressing)
- Additional olive oil for dressing (1-2 tablespoons)

Instructions

1. Prepare the Chicken: Season the chicken breasts with olive oil, salt, pepper, and garlic powder (if using). Grill the chicken over medium-high heat for about 6-7 minutes on each side or until fully cooked and the internal temperature reaches 165°F (74°C). Remove from the grill and let it rest for a few minutes before slicing.
2. Assemble the Salad: In a large salad bowl, combine the mixed greens, diced avocado, cherry tomatoes, cucumber, and red onion (if using). Toss gently to mix the ingredients.
3. Add the Chicken: Slice the grilled chicken and arrange it on top of the salad.
4. Dress the Salad: Drizzle the lemon juice and additional olive oil over the salad. Toss gently to combine.
5. Serve: Enjoy your refreshing salad immediately!

1 serving (approximately 1 large bowl)

Nutritional Information (Approximate per serving)

- Calories: 400

- Protein: 30g

- Fat: 28g

- Carbohydrates: 12g

- Fiber: 8g

- Sugar: 2g

- Sodium: 360mg (varies based on added salt)

- Potassium: 800mg (23% DV)

- Phosphorus: 300mg (24% DV)

Why This Recipe is Good for Low-Lectin Dieters

The Grilled Chicken Salad with Avocado and Mixed Greens is an ideal choice for those following a low-lectin diet. Chicken is a lean protein source that is free from lectins, while mixed greens and avocado provide essential vitamins, minerals, and healthy fats without the negative effects associated with high-lectin foods. The use of fresh vegetables like cucumbers and tomatoes adds flavor and nutrients, making this salad not only satisfying but also a powerhouse of health benefits. This recipe is perfect for lunch or dinner and can be easily customized to suit your preferences.

Quinoa Salad with Cucumber, Bell Pepper, and Olive Oil Dressing

Ingredients

- 1 cup quinoa (rinsed)
- 2 cups water or low-sodium vegetable broth
- 1 medium cucumber, diced
- 1 cup bell peppers, diced (any color)
- 1/4 red onion, finely chopped (optional)
- 1/4 cup fresh parsley, chopped
- 2 tablespoons olive oil
- 1 tablespoon lemon juice (freshly squeezed)
- Salt and pepper, to taste

Instructions

1. Cook the Quinoa: In a medium saucepan, bring 2 cups of water or broth to a boil. Add the rinsed quinoa and a pinch of salt. Reduce the heat to low, cover, and simmer for about 15 minutes, or until the quinoa is fluffy and the liquid is absorbed. Remove from heat and let it sit covered for 5 minutes, then fluff with a fork.
2. Prepare the Salad: In a large bowl, combine the cooked quinoa, diced cucumber, diced bell peppers, red onion (if using), and chopped parsley.
3. Make the Dressing: In a small bowl, whisk together the olive oil, lemon juice, salt, and pepper.
4. Combine: Pour the dressing over the salad and toss gently to combine all ingredients.
5. Serve: This salad can be served immediately or chilled in the refrigerator for 30 minutes to allow the flavors to meld. Enjoy!

1 serving (approximately 1.5 Cups)

Nutritional Information (Approximate per serving)

- Calories: 250

- Protein: 8g

- Fat: 12g

- Carbohydrates: 30g

- Fiber: 6g

- Sugar: 3g

- Sodium: 180mg (varies based on added salt and broth)

- Potassium: 450mg (13% DV)

- Phosphorus: 150mg (12% DV)

Why This Recipe is Good for Low-Lectin Dieters

This Quinoa Salad with Cucumber, Bell Pepper, and Olive Oil Dressing is an excellent choice for those following a low-lectin diet. Quinoa is a versatile grain that is relatively low in lectins compared to other grains and is a complete protein, making it a nutritious addition to any meal. The fresh vegetables add essential vitamins, minerals, and hydration without the negative effects of high-lectin foods. The olive oil dressing provides healthy fats that promote satiety and overall health. This salad is not only refreshing and satisfying but also a perfect option for lunch or as a side dish.

Zucchini Noodles with Marinara Sauce and Grilled Shrimp

Ingredients

For the Zucchini Noodles:
- 2 medium zucchinis, spiralized or sliced into thin noodles
- 1 tablespoon olive oil
- Salt and pepper, to taste
- 1/2 teaspoon garlic powder (optional)

For the Marinara Sauce:
- 1 can (14.5 oz) crushed tomatoes (no salt added)
- 2 cloves garlic, minced
- 1 small onion, finely chopped
- 1 teaspoon dried oregano
- 1 teaspoon dried basil
- 1 tablespoon olive oil
- Salt and pepper, to taste

For the Grilled Shrimp:
- 1 pound large shrimp, peeled and deveined
- 2 tablespoons olive oil
- 1 teaspoon paprika (optional)
- Salt and pepper, to taste
- 1 tablespoon lemon juice (optional, for added flavor)

Instructions

1. Prepare the Marinara Sauce:
2. In a medium saucepan, heat 1 tablespoon of olive oil over medium heat. Add the chopped onion and sauté for about 3-4 minutes until the onion becomes translucent.
3. Add the minced garlic and cook for an additional minute until fragrant.
4. Stir in the crushed tomatoes, oregano, basil, salt, and pepper. Bring the sauce to a simmer and let it cook for about 10-15 minutes to allow the flavors to meld.
5. Grill the Shrimp:
6. In a bowl, toss the shrimp with olive oil, paprika (if using), salt, and pepper. Preheat a grill or grill pan over medium-high heat.
7. Grill the shrimp for about 2-3 minutes on each side, or until they are pink and opaque. Drizzle with lemon juice before removing from the grill.
8. Cook the Zucchini Noodles:
9. In a large skillet, heat 1 tablespoon of olive oil over medium heat. Add the zucchini noodles and sauté for about 2-3 minutes, or until they are tender but still have a slight crunch. Season with salt, pepper, and garlic powder (if using).

	10. Combine and Serve:
	11. To serve, place the zucchini noodles on a plate, top with marinara sauce, and add the grilled shrimp on top. Garnish with fresh basil or parsley if desired.
1 serving (approximately 1.5 Cups)	

Nutritional Information (Approximate per serving)

- Calories: 350

- Protein: 28g

- Fat: 20g

- Carbohydrates: 15g

- Fiber: 4g

- Sugar: 6g

- Sodium: 400mg (varies based on added salt)

- Potassium: 700mg (20% DV)

- Phosphorus: 250mg (20% DV)

Why This Recipe is Good for Low-Lectin Dieters

Zucchini Noodles with Marinara Sauce and Grilled Shrimp is an excellent low-lectin meal that combines the benefits of fresh vegetables and lean protein. Zucchini is low in lectins and provides a nutritious alternative to traditional pasta, while the shrimp offers a rich source of protein without any lectins. The homemade marinara sauce, made from crushed tomatoes and herbs, is flavorful and free from high-lectin ingredients. This dish is not only delicious and satisfying but also supports a healthy lifestyle by minimizing lectin intake.

Baked Salmon with Lemon and Herbs, Served with Asparagus

Ingredients	Instructions
For the Salmon: • 2 salmon fillets (about 6 oz each) • 2 tablespoons olive oil • 1 lemon, sliced • 2 teaspoons fresh dill or 1 teaspoon dried dill (or other herbs like thyme or parsley) • Salt and pepper, to taste **For the Asparagus:** • 1 bunch asparagus, trimmed • 1 tablespoon olive oil • Salt and pepper, to taste • 1 lemon wedge (for serving)	1. Preheat the Oven: Preheat your oven to 400°F (200°C). 2. Prepare the Salmon: Place the salmon fillets on a baking sheet lined with parchment paper. Drizzle with olive oil and season with salt, pepper, and dill. Top each fillet with lemon slices. 3. Prepare the Asparagus: In a separate bowl, toss the trimmed asparagus with olive oil, salt, and pepper. Arrange the asparagus on the same baking sheet as the salmon, placing it around the fillets. 4. Bake: Place the baking sheet in the preheated oven and bake for about 15-20 minutes, or until the salmon flakes easily with a fork and the asparagus is tender. 5. Serve: Remove from the oven and serve the salmon and asparagus warm, with a squeeze of fresh lemon juice over the top if desired.

1 serving (approximately 1 salmon fillet and 1 cup of asparagus)

Nutritional Information (Approximate per serving)

- Calories: 350

- Protein: 30g

- Fat: 22g

- Carbohydrates: 8g

- Fiber: 4g

- Sugar: 2g

- Sodium: 300mg (varies based on added salt)

- Potassium: 800mg (23% DV)

- Phosphorus: 300mg (24% DV)

Why This Recipe is Good for Low-Lectin Dieters

Baked Salmon with Lemon and Herbs, Served with Asparagus is an ideal dish for those following a low-lectin diet. Salmon is a rich source of omega-3 fatty acids and high-quality protein, with no lectins, making it a heart-healthy choice. Asparagus is low in lectins and provides essential vitamins and minerals, along with dietary fiber. The combination of fresh herbs and lemon not only enhances the flavors but also adds additional nutrients without introducing high-lectin ingredients. This dish is both nutritious and satisfying, making it perfect for lunch or dinner.

Stuffed Bell Peppers with Ground Turkey and Cauliflower Rice

Ingredients

For the Stuffed Peppers:

- 4 large bell peppers (any color)
- 1 pound ground turkey (lean)
- 2 cups cauliflower rice (fresh or frozen cauliflower processed into rice-sized pieces)
- 1 small onion, finely chopped
- 2 cloves garlic, minced
- 1 can (14.5 oz) diced tomatoes, no salt added
- 1 teaspoon dried oregano
- 1 teaspoon dried basil
- Salt and pepper, to taste
- 1 tablespoon olive oil
- 1/2 cup shredded cheese (optional; such as mozzarella or cheddar)
- Fresh parsley, chopped (for garnish)

Instructions

1. Preheat the Oven: Preheat your oven to 375°F (190°C).
2. Prepare the Bell Peppers: Cut the tops off the bell peppers and remove the seeds and membranes. If necessary, trim the bottoms slightly to ensure they stand upright. Place the peppers in a baking dish, cut side up.
3. Cook the Filling:
4. In a large skillet, heat 1 tablespoon of olive oil over medium heat. Add the chopped onion and garlic, and sauté for about 3-4 minutes until the onion is translucent.
5. Add the ground turkey to the skillet, breaking it apart with a spoon. Cook until browned and fully cooked, about 5-7 minutes.
6. Stir in the cauliflower rice, diced tomatoes (with their juices), oregano, basil, salt, and pepper. Cook for another 2-3 minutes until everything is heated through.
7. Stuff the Peppers: Spoon the turkey and cauliflower rice mixture into each bell pepper, packing it down gently. If desired, sprinkle shredded cheese on top of each stuffed pepper.
8. Bake: Cover the baking dish with aluminum foil and bake in the preheated oven for 25-30

	minutes. Remove the foil during the last 10 minutes of baking to allow the cheese to melt and the tops to brown slightly.
	9. Serve: Once cooked, remove from the oven and let cool for a few minutes. Garnish with fresh parsley before serving.
1 serving (approximately 1 stuffed bell pepper)	

Nutritional Information (Approximate per serving)

- Calories: 290
- Protein: 28g
- Fat: 12g
- Carbohydrates: 18g
- Fiber: 5g
- Sugar: 4g
- Sodium: 320mg (varies based on added salt and cheese)
- Potassium: 600mg (17% DV)
- Phosphorus: 250mg (20% DV)

Why This Recipe is Good for Low-Lectin Dieters

Stuffed Bell Peppers with Ground Turkey and Cauliflower Rice is an excellent choice for those following a low-lectin diet. Ground turkey is a lean protein source that is low in lectins, while bell peppers and cauliflower are both low-lectin vegetables packed with vitamins and minerals. This dish not only provides a satisfying and nutritious meal but also incorporates a variety of flavors and textures, making it enjoyable for everyone. Additionally, it can be easily customized with different herbs and spices to suit your taste.

Slow-Cooked Chicken Thighs with Garlic and Rosemary

Ingredients

- 4 bone-in, skin-on chicken thighs (about 1.5 lbs)
- 4 cloves garlic, minced
- 2 tablespoons fresh rosemary, chopped (or 1 tablespoon dried rosemary)
- 1 tablespoon olive oil
- 1 cup low-sodium chicken broth
- Salt and pepper, to taste
- 1 lemon, sliced (for garnish)

Instructions

1. Prepare the Chicken: Season the chicken thighs generously with salt and pepper on both sides.
2. Sauté the Garlic: In a skillet, heat the olive oil over medium heat. Add the minced garlic and sauté for about 1 minute until fragrant but not browned.
3. Brown the Chicken (Optional): If desired, you can brown the chicken thighs in the skillet for 3-4 minutes on each side until golden brown. This step adds flavor but can be skipped if you're short on time.
4. Transfer to Slow Cooker: Place the browned (or raw) chicken thighs in the slow cooker. Sprinkle the chopped rosemary over the top, then pour in the low-sodium chicken broth.
5. Cook: Cover the slow cooker and cook on low for 6-7 hours or on high for 3-4 hours, until the chicken is tender and fully cooked.
6. Serve: Once cooked, remove the chicken thighs from the slow cooker and let them rest for a few minutes. Serve warm, garnished with lemon slices.

1 serving (approximately 1 chicken thigh with sauce)

Nutritional Information (Approximate per serving)

- Calories: 320

- Protein: 25g

- Fat: 22g

- Carbohydrates: 2g

- Fiber: 0g

- Sugar: 0g

- Sodium: 350mg (varies based on added salt and broth)

- Potassium: 500mg (14% DV)

- Phosphorus: 220mg (18% DV)

Why This Recipe is Good for Low-Lectin Dieters

Slow-Cooked Chicken Thighs with Garlic and Rosemary is a fantastic option for those following a low-lectin diet. Chicken thighs are a rich source of protein without any lectins, making them an excellent choice for a satisfying meal. The garlic and rosemary not only add delicious flavor but also provide antioxidant and anti-inflammatory properties. Slow cooking ensures that the chicken remains tender and flavorful, while the low-sodium broth keeps the dish heart-healthy. This recipe is easy to prepare and perfect for busy weeknights, allowing you to enjoy a nutritious, low-lectin meal with minimal effort.

Cucumber and Bell Pepper Sticks with Hummus

Ingredients

For the Vegetable Sticks:
- 1 medium cucumber, cut into sticks
- 1 large bell pepper (any color), cut into sticks
- 1 cup carrot sticks (optional, for added variety)

For the Hummus:
- 1 can (15 oz) chickpeas, drained and rinsed
- 2 tablespoons tahini
- 2 tablespoons olive oil
- 1 clove garlic, minced
- 2 tablespoons lemon juice (freshly squeezed)
- Salt and pepper, to taste
- Water, as needed for consistency

Instructions

1. Prepare the Vegetable Sticks: Wash and cut the cucumber and bell pepper into sticks. If using, cut the carrots into sticks as well. Arrange them on a platter or in individual serving cups.
2. Make the Hummus: In a food processor, combine the drained chickpeas, tahini, olive oil, minced garlic, lemon juice, salt, and pepper. Blend until smooth. If the mixture is too thick, add water a tablespoon at a time until you reach your desired consistency.
3. Serve: Transfer the hummus to a serving bowl and serve alongside the prepared vegetable sticks. Enjoy as a healthy snack or appetizer!

1 serving (approximately 1 cup of vegetable sticks with 1/4 cup of hummus)

Nutritional Information (Approximate per serving, 1 cup vegetable sticks with 1/4 cup hummus)

- Calories: 150
- Protein: 5g
- Fat: 8g
- Carbohydrates: 18g
- Fiber: 5g
- Sugar: 3g
- Sodium: 200mg (varies based on added salt)
- Potassium: 400mg (11% DV)
- Phosphorus: 150mg (12% DV)

Why This Recipe is Good for Low-Lectin Dieters

Cucumber and Bell Pepper Sticks with Hummus is an excellent choice for those following a low-lectin diet. The fresh vegetables are low in lectins and provide essential vitamins, minerals, and hydration. Cucumber and bell pepper are particularly rich in Vitamin C, supporting immune health and skin integrity. Hummus, made from chickpeas, offers a good source of plant-based protein and healthy fats. This recipe is not only nutritious but also quick and easy to prepare, making it a perfect snack or appetizer that fits well within a low-lectin lifestyle.

Rice Cakes with Almond Butter and Sliced Strawberries

Ingredients

- 4 plain rice cakes (ensure they are low sodium and gluten-free, if needed)
- 1/2 cup almond butter (natural, no added sugar or salt)
- 1 cup fresh strawberries, hulled and sliced
- 1 tablespoon honey (optional, for added sweetness)
- Chia seeds or cinnamon (optional, for garnish)

Instructions

1. Prepare the Strawberries: Wash and hull the strawberries, then slice them into thin rounds.
2. Spread Almond Butter: Take each rice cake and spread a generous layer of almond butter on top.
3. Add Strawberries: Arrange the sliced strawberries on top of the almond butter-covered rice cakes. If desired, drizzle a little honey over the strawberries for added sweetness.
4. Garnish: If using, sprinkle with chia seeds or a dash of cinnamon for extra flavor and nutrition.
5. Serve: Enjoy immediately as a healthy snack or light meal!

1 serving (approximately 2 Rice Cakes)

Nutritional Information (Approximate per serving, 2 rice cakes)

- Calories: 300

- Protein: 10g

- Fat: 20g

- Carbohydrates: 30g

- Fiber: 6g

- Sugar: 8g (from strawberries and honey)

- Sodium: 150mg (varies based on rice cakes)

- Potassium: 400mg (11% DV)

- Phosphorus: 150mg (12% DV)

Why This Recipe is Good for Low-Lectin Dieters

Rice Cakes with Almond Butter and Sliced Strawberries is an ideal snack for those following a low-lectin diet. Rice cakes are generally low in lectins and provide a light, crunchy base. Almond butter adds healthy fats and protein without the complications that come with high-lectin foods. The fresh strawberries are not only delicious but also rich in Vitamin C and antioxidants, making this snack nutritious and satisfying. This recipe is quick to prepare and perfect for any time of day, whether as a snack or a light breakfast.

Hard-Boiled Eggs with Avocado and Sea Salt

Ingredients

- 4 large eggs
- 1 ripe avocado, halved and pitted
- Sea salt, to taste
- Freshly ground black pepper (optional)
- Red pepper flakes or paprika (optional for garnish)
- Lemon juice (optional, for drizzling)

Instructions

1. Boil the Eggs: Place the eggs in a saucepan and cover them with cold water. Bring the water to a boil over medium-high heat. Once boiling, cover the pan and remove it from heat. Let the eggs sit in the hot water for about 9-12 minutes, depending on how well-done you prefer your yolks.
2. Cool the Eggs: After the time is up, transfer the eggs to a bowl of ice water or run them under cold water for a few minutes to stop the cooking process. Once cooled, peel the eggs.
3. Prepare the Avocado: While the eggs are cooling, slice the avocado in half. Remove the pit and scoop out the avocado flesh into a small bowl. Mash it lightly with a fork, or leave it chunky, depending on your preference.
4. Assemble: Slice the hard-boiled eggs in half and place them on a plate. Top each egg half with a spoonful of mashed avocado.
5. Season: Sprinkle with sea salt and freshly ground black pepper to taste. If desired, drizzle with a little lemon juice and garnish with red pepper flakes or paprika for an extra kick.
6. Serve: Enjoy immediately as a nutritious snack or light meal!

1 serving (approximately 2 egg halves with avocado)

Nutritional Information (Approximate per serving, 2 egg halves with avocado)

- Calories: 250

- Protein: 12g

- Fat: 20g

- Carbohydrates: 12g

- Fiber: 6g

- Sugar: 1g

- Sodium: 180mg (varies based on added salt)

- Potassium: 550mg (16% DV)

- Phosphorus: 200mg (16% DV)

Why This Recipe is Good for Low-Lectin Dieters

Hard-Boiled Eggs with Avocado and Sea Salt is an excellent option for those on a low-lectin diet. Eggs are a fantastic source of high-quality protein and contain no lectins, making them a staple for many health-conscious individuals. Avocado is rich in heart-healthy fats and fiber, providing essential nutrients without the negative effects associated with high-lectin foods. This recipe is simple, quick to prepare, and incredibly satisfying, making it a perfect snack or light meal that aligns with low-lectin dietary principles.

DESSERT RECIPES

Hard-Boiled Eggs with Avocado and Sea Salt

Ingredients

- 1 cup almond butter (natural, no added sugar or salt)
- 1/4 cup honey or maple syrup
- 1 large egg
- 1 teaspoon vanilla extract
- 1/2 teaspoon baking soda
- 1/4 teaspoon salt (optional)
- 1/2 cup dark chocolate chips (ensure they are low in sugar and suitable for low-lectin diets)

Instructions

1. Preheat the Oven: Preheat your oven to 350°F (175°C) and line a baking sheet with parchment paper.
2. Mix Ingredients: In a large mixing bowl, combine the almond butter, honey (or maple syrup), egg, vanilla extract, baking soda, and salt (if using). Stir until the mixture is smooth and well combined.
3. Add Chocolate Chips: Fold in the dark chocolate chips until evenly distributed throughout the dough.
4. Shape the Cookies: Using a tablespoon or cookie scoop, drop rounded balls of dough onto the prepared baking sheet, spacing them about 2 inches apart. Flatten each ball slightly with the back of a fork or your fingers.
5. Bake: Bake in the preheated oven for about 10-12 minutes, or until the edges are golden brown.
6. Cool and Serve: Remove from the oven and let the cookies cool on the baking sheet for a few minutes before transferring them to a wire rack to cool completely.

1 serving (approximately 2 cookies)

Nutritional Information (Approximate per serving, 2 cookies)

- Calories: 220

- Protein: 6g

- Fat: 14g

- Carbohydrates: 24g

- Fiber: 3g

- Sugar: 8g (from honey/maple syrup and chocolate chips)

- Sodium: 150mg (varies based on added salt)

- Potassium: 200mg (6% DV)

- Phosphorus: 150mg (12% DV)

Why This Recipe is Good for Low-Lectin Dieters

Almond Butter Cookies with Dark Chocolate Chips are an excellent choice for those following a low-lectin diet. Almond butter is low in lectins and provides healthy fats and protein, making it a nutritious base for cookies. The addition of dark chocolate chips adds sweetness and antioxidants without compromising the low-lectin principles. This recipe is not only delicious but also offers a satisfying treat that aligns with your dietary goals, making it a great option for snacks or dessert.

Baked Apples with Cinnamon and Walnuts

Ingredients

- 4 medium apples (such as Fuji or Gala), cored
- 1/2 cup walnuts, chopped
- 1/4 cup raisins (optional, for added sweetness)
- 1 teaspoon cinnamon
- 2 tablespoons honey or maple syrup (optional, adjust sweetness to taste)
- 1 tablespoon butter or coconut oil (for greasing)
- 1/2 cup water (for baking)

Instructions

1. Preheat the Oven: Preheat your oven to 350°F (175°C).
2. Prepare the Apples: Core the apples, making sure to leave the bottom intact to hold the filling. Place the apples upright in a baking dish.
3. Make the Filling: In a bowl, combine the chopped walnuts, raisins (if using), cinnamon, and honey (if using). Mix until well combined.
4. Stuff the Apples: Spoon the walnut mixture into the cored apples, packing it down gently.
5. Add Water: Pour the water into the bottom of the baking dish to help steam the apples as they bake, preventing them from drying out.
6. Bake: Cover the baking dish with aluminum foil and bake in the preheated oven for about 25-30 minutes, or until the apples are tender but still hold their shape.
7. Serve: Remove from the oven and let cool slightly. Serve warm, drizzled with any remaining juices from the baking dish.

1 serving (approximately 1 Baked Apple)

Nutritional Information (Approximate per serving, 1 baked apple)

- Calories: 180

- Protein: 2g

- Fat: 7g

- Carbohydrates: 30g

- Fiber: 4g

- Sugar: 15g (from apples and honey)

- Sodium: 5mg (varies based on added salt)

- Potassium: 200mg (6% DV)

- Phosphorus: 60mg (5% DV)

Why This Recipe is Good for Low-Lectin Dieters

Baked Apples with Cinnamon and Walnuts is a delightful dessert that fits perfectly within a low-lectin diet. Apples are naturally low in lectins and provide a good source of fiber, vitamins, and antioxidants. Walnuts add healthy fats and additional protein, making this dish both satisfying and nutritious. The warming spices of cinnamon enhance the flavor profile while offering anti-inflammatory benefits. This recipe is simple to prepare and can be enjoyed as a comforting dessert that aligns with your dietary goals.

Coconut Macaroons with a Drizzle of Dark Chocolate

Ingredients

- 2 1/2 cups shredded unsweetened coconut
- 1/2 cup sweetened condensed milk
- 1 teaspoon vanilla extract
- 2 large egg whites
- 1/4 teaspoon salt
- 1/2 cup dark chocolate chips (for drizzling)

Instructions

1. Preheat the Oven: Preheat your oven to 325°F (165°C) and line a baking sheet with parchment paper.
2. Mix Ingredients: In a large bowl, combine the shredded coconut, sweetened condensed milk, and vanilla extract. Stir until well mixed.
3. Whisk Egg Whites: In a separate bowl, whisk the egg whites and salt until soft peaks form (about 2-3 minutes with an electric mixer).
4. Fold Egg Whites: Gently fold the whipped egg whites into the coconut mixture until just combined. Be careful not to deflate the egg whites too much.
5. Form Macaroons: Using a tablespoon or a cookie scoop, drop heaping spoonfuls of the mixture onto the prepared baking sheet, spacing them about 1 inch apart.
6. Bake: Bake in the preheated oven for about 20-25 minutes, or until the tops are golden brown.
7. Cool: Remove from the oven and let the macaroons cool on the baking sheet for a few minutes before transferring them to a wire rack to cool completely.
8. Melt Chocolate: While the macaroons cool, melt the dark chocolate chips in a microwave-safe bowl or over a double boiler until smooth.

	9. Drizzle: Once the macaroons are cool, drizzle the melted chocolate over the tops using a fork or a piping bag. 10. Serve: Allow the chocolate to set before serving. Enjoy your delicious coconut macaroons!
	1 serving (approximately 2 Macaroons)

Nutritional Information (Approximate per serving, 2 macaroons)

- Calories: 220
- Protein: 3g
- Fat: 15g
- Carbohydrates: 24g
- Fiber: 3g
- Sugar: 12g (from condensed milk and chocolate)
- Sodium: 50mg (varies based on added salt)
- Potassium: 150mg (4% DV)
- Phosphorus: 100mg (8% DV)

Why This Recipe is Good for Low-Lectin Dieters

Coconut Macaroons with a Drizzle of Dark Chocolate are a delightful treat for those on a low-lectin diet. Shredded coconut is low in lectins and provides healthy fats, fiber, and a natural sweetness that satisfies cravings without adding high-lectin ingredients. The use of egg whites helps bind the macaroons while adding protein without the lectins found in many other binding agents. Dark chocolate adds a rich flavor and antioxidants, making this dessert not only indulgent but also aligned with your health goals. This recipe is perfect for satisfying your sweet tooth while adhering to a low-lectin lifestyle.

Cauliflower Rice Stir-Fry with Mixed Vegetables and Chicken

Ingredients

- 1 pound boneless, skinless chicken breasts, cut into bite-sized pieces
- 1 medium head of cauliflower, grated or processed into rice-sized pieces (about 4 cups)
- 2 tablespoons vegetable oil (such as canola or sesame oil)
- 2 cloves garlic, minced
- 1 small onion, chopped
- 1 cup bell peppers, diced (any color)
- 1 cup broccoli florets
- 1 cup snap peas or green beans, trimmed
- 2 tablespoons low-sodium soy sauce (or tamari for gluten-free)
- 1 tablespoon sesame oil (optional, for flavor)
- Salt and pepper, to taste
- Green onions, sliced (for garnish)

Instructions

1. Prepare the Cauliflower Rice: Remove the leaves and stem from the cauliflower, and cut it into florets. Use a food processor to pulse the florets until they resemble rice-sized grains. Alternatively, you can grate the cauliflower using a box grater.
2. Cook the Chicken: In a large skillet or wok, heat the vegetable oil over medium-high heat. Add the chicken pieces and season with salt and pepper. Cook for about 5-7 minutes, or until the chicken is cooked through and golden brown. Remove the chicken from the skillet and set aside.
3. Sauté the Vegetables: In the same skillet, add the chopped onion and minced garlic. Sauté for about 2-3 minutes until the onion is translucent. Add the bell peppers, broccoli, and snap peas, and stir-fry for about 5 minutes until the vegetables are tender-crisp.
4. Add Cauliflower Rice: Stir in the cauliflower rice and soy sauce. Cook for an additional 5-7 minutes, stirring frequently, until the cauliflower is tender and heated through. Return the cooked chicken to the skillet and mix well.

	5. Finish with Seasoning: Drizzle with sesame oil (if using) and adjust seasoning with salt and pepper to taste. Toss to combine.
	6. Serve: Remove from heat and garnish with sliced green onions. Serve warm as a main dish.
1 serving (approximately 1.5 Cups)	

Nutritional Information (Approximate per serving)

- Calories: 300
- Protein: 30g
- Fat: 14g
- Carbohydrates: 16g
- Fiber: 5g
- Sugar: 3g
- Sodium: 400mg (varies based on added salt and soy sauce)
- Potassium: 600mg (17% DV)
- Phosphorus: 250mg (20% DV)

Why This Recipe is Good for Low-Lectin Dieters

Cauliflower Rice Stir-Fry with Mixed Vegetables and Chicken is an excellent choice for those following a low-lectin diet. Cauliflower rice serves as a low-lectin alternative to traditional rice, providing a low-carb, nutrient-rich base for the stir-fry. Chicken is a lean protein source that is free from lectins, while the variety of vegetables adds essential vitamins, minerals, and fiber without the negative effects associated with high-lectin foods. This dish is not only quick and easy to prepare but also packed with flavor and nutrition, making it a satisfying and healthy meal option.

Vegetable Soup with Low Lectin Ingredients

Ingredients

- 1 tablespoon olive oil
- 1 medium onion, chopped
- 2 cloves garlic, minced
- 2 medium carrots, diced
- 1 medium zucchini, diced
- 1 bell pepper (any color), diced
- 1 cup cauliflower florets
- 1 cup green beans, trimmed and cut into pieces
- 4 cups low-sodium vegetable broth
- 1 can (14.5 oz) diced tomatoes, no salt added
- 1 teaspoon dried thyme
- 1 teaspoon dried basil
- Salt and pepper, to taste
- 1 cup kale or Swiss chard leaves, chopped (optional, used in moderation)
- Fresh parsley, chopped (for garnish)

Instructions

1. Sauté the Vegetables: In a large pot, heat the olive oil over medium heat. Add the chopped onion and garlic, and sauté for about 3-4 minutes until the onion is translucent.
2. Add Carrots and Zucchini: Stir in the diced carrots and zucchini, and cook for another 3-4 minutes.
3. Add Remaining Vegetables: Add the diced bell pepper, cauliflower florets, green beans, vegetable broth, diced tomatoes (with their juices), thyme, and basil. Stir to combine.
4. Simmer the Soup: Bring the soup to a boil, then reduce the heat to low. Cover and let it simmer for about 20-25 minutes, or until the vegetables are tender. If using kale or Swiss chard, add it in the last 5 minutes of cooking.
5. Season: Taste the soup and adjust the seasoning with salt and pepper as needed.
6. Serve: Ladle the soup into bowls and garnish with fresh parsley. Enjoy hot!

1 serving (approximately 1.5 Cups)

Nutritional Information (Approximate per serving)

- Calories: 120
- Protein: 4g
- Fat: 4g
- Carbohydrates: 18g
- Fiber: 5g
- Sugar: 4g
- Sodium: 200mg (varies based on broth used)
- Potassium: 600mg (17% DV)
- Phosphorus: 70mg (6% DV)

Why This Recipe is Good for Low-Lectin Dieters

Vegetable Soup with Low Lectin Ingredients is an excellent choice for those following a low-lectin diet. The variety of vegetables used in this soup are low in lectins and provide a rich source of vitamins, minerals, and antioxidants. This soup is not only comforting and nourishing but also packed with fiber, which supports digestive health. Additionally, it is easy to customize based on seasonal vegetables or personal preferences, making it a versatile and healthful option that fits well within a low-lectin lifestyle.

Egg Muffins with Spinach and Cheese

Ingredients

- 6 large eggs
- 1 cup fresh spinach, chopped
- 1/2 cup shredded cheese (such as cheddar or mozzarella)
- 1/4 cup milk (dairy or non-dairy, unsweetened)
- 1/4 teaspoon salt (or to taste)
- 1/4 teaspoon black pepper (or to taste)
- 1/4 teaspoon garlic powder (optional)
- 1/4 cup diced bell pepper (optional)

Instructions

1. Preheat the Oven: Preheat your oven to 350°F (175°C) and grease a muffin tin with cooking spray or olive oil.
2. Prepare the Egg Mixture: In a large bowl, whisk together the eggs, milk, salt, pepper, and garlic powder (if using) until well combined.
3. Add Vegetables and Cheese: Stir in the chopped spinach, diced bell pepper (if using), and shredded cheese. Mix until evenly distributed.
4. Fill the Muffin Tin: Pour the egg mixture into the prepared muffin tin, filling each cup about 2/3 full.
5. Bake: Bake in the preheated oven for about 18-20 minutes, or until the muffins are set and lightly golden on top. You can check for doneness by inserting a toothpick in the center; it should come out clean.
6. Cool and Serve: Allow the egg muffins to cool in the pan for a few minutes before gently removing them. Serve warm or at room temperature.

1 serving (approximately 2 Egg Muffins)

Nutritional Information (Approximate per serving, 2 muffins)

- Calories: 180

- Protein: 12g

- Fat: 12g

- Carbohydrates: 2g

- Fiber: 1g

- Sugar: 1g

- Sodium: 320mg (varies based on added salt and cheese)

- Potassium: 300mg (9% DV)

- Phosphorus: 200mg (16% DV)

Why This Recipe is Good for Low-Lectin Dieters

Egg Muffins with Spinach and Cheese are an excellent option for those following a low-lectin diet. Eggs are a fantastic source of high-quality protein with no lectins, while spinach adds essential vitamins and minerals without the negative effects associated with high-lectin foods. The addition of cheese provides flavor and healthy fats, making these muffins both satisfying and nutritious. They are also convenient for meal prep, as they can be made in advance and enjoyed throughout the week, making them a perfect grab-and-go breakfast or snack option.

Grilled Zucchini and Eggplant with Olive Oil and Herbs

Ingredients

- 2 medium zucchinis, sliced into 1/4-inch rounds
- 1 medium eggplant, sliced into 1/4-inch rounds
- 3 tablespoons olive oil
- 1 teaspoon dried oregano
- 1 teaspoon dried thyme
- Salt and pepper, to taste
- 1 tablespoon balsamic vinegar (optional, for added flavor)
- Fresh herbs (such as basil or parsley) for garnish

Instructions

1. Preheat the Grill: Preheat your grill or grill pan over medium-high heat.
2. Prepare the Vegetables: In a large bowl, combine the sliced zucchini and eggplant. Drizzle with olive oil, and sprinkle with oregano, thyme, salt, and pepper. Toss until the vegetables are evenly coated.
3. Grill the Vegetables: Place the zucchini and eggplant slices on the grill. Grill for about 4-5 minutes on each side, or until they are tender and have nice grill marks.
4. Add Balsamic Vinegar: If using, drizzle the grilled vegetables with balsamic vinegar just before removing them from the grill for added flavor.
5. Serve: Transfer the grilled zucchini and eggplant to a serving platter and garnish with fresh herbs. Serve warm or at room temperature.

1 serving (approximately 1 Cup of Grilled Vegetables)

Nutritional Information (Approximate per serving)

- Calories: 120

- Protein: 3g

- Fat: 10g

- Carbohydrates: 8g

- Fiber: 4g

- Sugar: 3g

- Sodium: 250mg (varies based on added salt)

- Potassium: 400mg (11% DV)

- Phosphorus: 50mg (4% DV)

Why This Recipe is Good for Low-Lectin Dieters

Grilled Zucchini and Eggplant with Olive Oil and Herbs is an excellent choice for those following a low-lectin diet. Both zucchini and eggplant are low in lectins and provide a wealth of vitamins, minerals, and antioxidants. Grilling enhances their natural flavors while minimizing the need for added ingredients that might contain lectins. The use of olive oil not only adds healthy fats but also provides anti-inflammatory benefits. This dish is not only delicious and satisfying but also versatile, serving as a great side dish or a light main course that aligns perfectly with low-lectin dietary principles.

Berry Parfait with Greek Yogurt and Honey

Ingredients

- 1 cup Greek yogurt (plain, low-fat or full-fat)
- 1/2 cup mixed berries (such as blueberries, strawberries, and raspberries)
- 2 tablespoons honey (or maple syrup for a different flavor)
- 1/4 cup low-lectin granola (optional)
- 1 tablespoon chia seeds (optional, for added fiber and omega-3s)
- Fresh mint leaves (optional, for garnish)

Instructions

1. Prepare the Berries: If using whole strawberries, slice them into smaller pieces. Rinse the berries under cold water and drain well.
2. Layer the Parfait: In a tall glass or bowl, start by adding a layer of Greek yogurt (about 1/3 cup).
3. Add Berries: Next, add a layer of mixed berries (about 1/4 cup) on top of the yogurt.
4. Drizzle Honey: Drizzle 1 tablespoon of honey over the berries.
5. Add Granola: Sprinkle a layer of granola (about 2 tablespoons) over the honey.
6. Repeat Layers: Repeat the layers one more time, starting with Greek yogurt, then berries, honey, and granola.
7. Finish and Serve: Top the parfait with a sprinkle of chia seeds (if using) and garnish with fresh mint leaves. Serve immediately.

1 serving (approximately 1 Cup)

Nutritional Information (Approximate per serving)

- Calories: 300

- Protein: 15g

- Fat: 8g

- Carbohydrates: 45g

- Fiber: 5g

- Sugar: 20g (from honey and berries)

- Sodium: 75mg (varies based on yogurt and granola used)

- Potassium: 400mg (11% DV)

- Phosphorus: 250mg (20% DV)

Why This Recipe is Good for Low-Lectin Dieters

The Berry Parfait with Greek Yogurt and Honey is an excellent choice for those following a low-lectin diet. Greek yogurt is a great source of protein and probiotics, promoting gut health without the lectins found in many dairy products. The mixed berries are low in lectins and rich in antioxidants and vitamins, particularly Vitamin C, which supports immune health. This parfait is not only delicious but also provides a satisfying and nutritious option for breakfast or a snack, making it a perfect addition to a low-lectin lifestyle.

122

Chapter 8: Shopping Made Simple

One-Week Shopping List

To help you get started with your low lectin meal plan, here's a comprehensive one-week shopping list based on the meals outlined in Chapter 6. This list includes all the ingredients you'll need, organized by category to make your shopping experience efficient.

CATEGORY	ITEMS
Fruits	Apples
	Blueberries
	Strawberries
	Bananas
	Lemons
	Kiwi
	Raspberries
Vegetables	Zucchini
	Cauliflower
	Broccoli
	Bell peppers (various colors)
	Spinach (cooked)
	Kale (cooked)
	Carrots
	Cucumbers
	Asparagus

	Green beans
	Mixed salad greens
Proteins	Ground turkey
	Chicken breasts
	Salmon fillets
	Eggs
	Firm tofu
Grains and Legumes	White rice
	Quinoa (in moderation)
	Rolled oats
Dairy and Dairy Alternatives	Greek yogurt (plain)
	Hard cheeses (e.g., cheddar, Parmesan)
	Almond milk (unsweetened)
	Coconut milk
Nuts and Seeds	Almonds
	Pecans
	Walnuts
	Chia seeds (optional)
Fats and Oils	Olive oil
	Coconut oil
	Avocado oil
Snacks and Sweets	Rice cakes
	Low lectin granola (optional)
	Dark chocolate chips (optional)

Tips for Shopping Low Lectin

When shopping for low lectin foods, consider the following tips to help you make informed choices:

1. *Read Labels:* Always check ingredient labels for hidden lectins and additives. Look for products that are specifically labeled as low lectin or free from high-lectin ingredients.

2. *Choose Fresh Over Processed*: Whenever possible, opt for fresh fruits and vegetables instead of canned or frozen versions, which may contain added sugars, salt, or preservatives that can increase lectin levels.

3. *Prioritize Whole Foods*: Focus on whole, unprocessed foods, which are typically lower in lectins and higher in nutrients. This includes fresh produce, lean proteins, and whole grains.

4. *Shop the Perimeter*: Most grocery stores have fresh produce, dairy, and meats located around the perimeter. Spend most of your shopping time in these sections to find healthier options.

5. *Plan Ahead*: Make your shopping list based on your meal plan to avoid impulse buys and ensure you have everything you need for the week.

6. *Buy in Bulk*: Consider buying staples like rice, oats, and quinoa in bulk to save money and reduce packaging waste.

7. *Stay Informed*: Familiarize yourself with the low lectin foods and ingredients to help you make better choices while shopping.

Where to Find Low Lectin Ingredients

Finding low lectin ingredients is becoming easier as awareness of dietary needs increases. Here are some places to look for low lectin foods:

1. Local Grocery Stores: Most supermarkets carry a wide range of fresh produce, dairy alternatives, and whole grains. Look for organic or specialty brands that may offer low lectin options.

2. Health Food Stores: Stores like Whole Foods or local health food shops often have a larger selection of specialty items, including low lectin snacks, gluten-free products, and organic produce.

3. Farmers' Markets: Visiting farmers' markets can provide access to fresh, local produce. Speak with farmers about their growing practices and choose low lectin fruits and vegetables.

4. Online Retailers: Websites like Amazon, Thrive Market, or specialty health food sites often sell low lectin products, including grains, snacks, and meal kits designed for specific dietary needs.

5. Ethnic Markets: Explore international grocery stores that may carry unique low lectin ingredients, such as different types of grains, spices, and fresh produce.

6. Community Supported Agriculture (CSA): Joining a CSA can provide you with fresh, seasonal produce directly from local farms, allowing you to choose low lectin options.

By following this shopping guide and utilizing these tips, you can simplify your grocery shopping experience while ensuring that you have all the ingredients necessary for a successful low lectin diet.

Chapter 9: Tips for Success

Navigating Social Situations and Dining Out

Adopting a low lectin diet can present unique challenges, especially when it comes to social situations or dining out. However, with some preparation and communication, you can enjoy these experiences without feeling overwhelmed by your dietary restrictions. Here are some strategies to help you navigate social gatherings and restaurant meals:

1. ***Communicate Your Needs:*** When invited to a gathering, don't hesitate to inform your host about your dietary preferences. Most people appreciate your openness and want to accommodate your needs. Offer to bring a low lectin dish to share, ensuring there's something safe for you to enjoy.

2. ***Research Restaurants:*** Before dining out, check the restaurant's menu online. Many establishments now provide nutritional information and ingredient lists, which can help you identify low lectin options. Look for restaurants that focus on fresh, whole foods, as they are more likely to accommodate dietary requests.

3. ***Ask Questions:*** When ordering at a restaurant, feel free to ask your server about how dishes are prepared and what ingredients are used. Inquire about low lectin options or modifications that can be made to a dish, such as substituting high-lectin ingredients with safer alternatives.

4. ***Choose Wisely:*** Opt for dishes that include grilled, baked, or steamed proteins and vegetables, as these cooking methods typically involve fewer high-lectin ingredients. Avoid sauces or dressings that may contain hidden lectins.

5. ***Portion Control:*** If you're unsure about the lectin content of certain foods, practice portion control. Enjoy smaller servings of higher lectin foods, paired with larger portions of low lectin options.

6. **Stay Positive:** Focus on the social aspects of dining out rather than solely on the food. Engage in conversations and enjoy the company of your friends and family, making the experience enjoyable regardless of the menu.

Involving Family in Meal Preparation

Involving family members in meal preparation can enhance your low lectin journey and create a supportive environment. Here are some ways to get your family involved:

1. **Educate Your Family:** Share information about the importance of a low lectin diet and how it benefits your health. When family members understand your dietary needs, they are more likely to support your choices.

2. **Plan Meals Together:** Encourage family involvement in meal planning. Sit down together to create a weekly meal plan that incorporates everyone's preferences while adhering to low lectin guidelines.

3. **Cook Together:** Make cooking a family activity. Involve kids and spouses in preparing meals, from washing vegetables to measuring ingredients. This not only fosters teamwork but also teaches valuable cooking skills.

4. **Experiment with Recipes:** Try new low lectin recipes as a family. Challenge each other to come up with creative dishes that everyone will enjoy. Use this opportunity to explore different cuisines and cooking techniques.

5. **Share Responsibilities:** Assign different family members specific meal preparation tasks, such as chopping vegetables, setting the table, or cleaning up afterward. Sharing responsibilities can make cooking less overwhelming and more enjoyable.

6. **Make it Fun:** Incorporate fun themes or challenges into your cooking sessions. For example, you could have a "low lectin taco night" where everyone assembles their own tacos with safe ingredients.

Staying Informed: Resources and Support Groups

Staying informed about the latest research, dietary guidelines, and support options can help you successfully manage your low lectin diet. Here are some resources and support groups to consider:

1. ***Books and Publications:*** Look for reputable books on low lectin diets or health. Some well-known titles include "The Plant Paradox" by Dr. Steven Gundry, which discusses the impact of lectins on health.

2. ***Online Resources:*** Websites such as the *Gundry MD* and other wellness blogs provide helpful information on low lectin diets, recipes, and tips for managing dietary changes.

3. ***Support Groups:*** Consider joining local or online support groups for individuals following a low lectin diet. These communities can offer encouragement, share experiences, and provide practical tips.

4. ***Registered Dietitians:*** Consulting with a registered dietitian who specializes in low lectin diets can provide personalized guidance tailored to your dietary needs. They can help you create meal plans, suggest safe food options, and address any nutritional concerns.

5. ***Social Media and Forums:*** Explore social media platforms and forums where individuals share their experiences with low lectin diets. Engaging with others facing similar challenges can provide motivation and new ideas for meals and recipes.

By implementing these tips for success, you can navigate social situations confidently, involve your family in your dietary journey, and stay informed about the best practices for managing a low lectin diet.

Chapter 10: Cultural Context and Personal Stories

The Importance of Family Meals in Low Lectin Dieting

Family meals have long been recognized as a cornerstone of cultural and social life. They provide an opportunity for connection, communication, and the sharing of traditions. In the context of a low lectin diet, family meals take on an even more significant role.

1. ***Creating a Supportive Environment:*** Family meals offer a chance to educate and involve loved ones in dietary choices. When everyone sits down together to enjoy a meal, it fosters a supportive environment where dietary preferences can be discussed openly. This is particularly important for those adopting a low lectin diet, as it can help alleviate feelings of isolation or frustration that may arise from eating differently.

2. ***Building New Traditions:*** Adopting a low lectin diet doesn't mean sacrificing the joy of shared meals. In fact, it can inspire new culinary traditions. Families can explore low lectin recipes together, creating dishes that everyone can enjoy. For example, making low lectin tacos with zucchini tortillas or preparing a hearty quinoa salad with grilled chicken can become exciting family activities that reinforce healthy eating habits.

3. ***Encouraging Healthy Choices:*** Sharing meals as a family encourages healthy eating patterns. Research shows that families who eat together tend to have better dietary habits, including increased fruit and vegetable consumption. By preparing and enjoying low lectin meals together, families can instill these habits in children and foster a lifelong appreciation for nutritious foods.

4. ***Celebrating Togetherness:*** Family meals are also an opportunity to celebrate milestones, holidays, and everyday moments. Incorporating low lectin foods into these gatherings can show that dietary changes can be enjoyable and delicious. Sharing recipes that highlight the flavors of low lectin ingredients can create a sense of community and connection around the dining table.

Personal Anecdotes from Caroline's Journey in Health Advocacy

As I reflect on my journey in health advocacy, I am reminded of how personal experiences have shaped my understanding of the importance of diet and nutrition.

Cooking with Family

One of my fondest memories is the time I gathered my family to create a low lectin feast for a holiday celebration. Instead of traditional dishes laden with high lectins, we collaborated on recipes that embraced wholesome, low lectin ingredients. My sons, Elijah and Isaac, took charge of making zucchini noodles, while I prepared a savory marinara sauce from fresh tomatoes and herbs. It was a joyful experience that not only brought us closer together but also reinforced the idea that healthy eating can be fun and inclusive.

—— o ——

Advocacy through Education

In my role as a nurse, I've often had the opportunity to educate patients about dietary changes that can improve their health outcomes. I recall a patient named Linda, who struggled with digestive issues and was feeling overwhelmed by conflicting dietary advice. After discussing the benefits of a low lectin diet, she decided to give it a try. I invited her to join a small cooking class I organized, where we prepared low lectin meals together. Seeing her confidence grow in the kitchen and her health improve was incredibly rewarding. It reinforced my belief that education and community support are vital for successful dietary changes.

—— o ——

Sharing My Journey

As I ventured further into the world of low lectin eating, I began sharing my recipes and experiences on social media. I was amazed by the positive response from my followers, many of whom were also navigating dietary restrictions. The sense of community that developed around our shared experiences was inspiring. It became clear that we were not just exchanging recipes; we were supporting one another in our health journeys.

These personal anecdotes highlight the profound impact that family, community, and shared meals can have on embracing a low lectin lifestyle. By creating an inclusive environment and encouraging open dialogue about dietary choices, we can help ourselves and others thrive in their health journeys.

Conclusion

Empowering Individuals to Manage Their Health

As we reach the end of The Complete Low Lectin Food List Guide, my hope is that you feel empowered and equipped to take charge of your health through informed dietary choices. Understanding the role of lectins in our diets and how they can impact our well-being is a significant step toward achieving optimal health.

This guide has provided you with comprehensive resources, including detailed food lists, practical meal planning strategies, and delicious recipes designed to help you navigate the low lectin lifestyle. Whether you are looking to alleviate digestive issues, reduce inflammation, or simply adopt a healthier way of eating, the information contained within these pages serves as a foundation for your journey.

Remember, dietary changes can take time and patience. It's essential to listen to your body and be open to experimentation. By focusing on whole, nutrient-dense foods and minimizing high-lectin ingredients, you can create a sustainable and enjoyable eating pattern that promotes overall health and vitality.

Recommendations for Low Lectin Dieting

While there may not be formal guidelines, the following general recommendations are commonly associated with a low lectin diet:

- Focus on Low Lectin Foods: Prioritize fruits, vegetables, healthy fats, and lean proteins while minimizing high-lectin foods.

- Preparation Methods: Cooking methods such as soaking, boiling, and fermenting can reduce lectin levels in foods like beans and grains.

- Listen to Your Body: Individual responses to lectins can vary, so it is essential to monitor how your body reacts to certain foods and adjust your diet accordingly.

- Consult Healthcare Professionals: It's advisable to work with a healthcare provider or registered dietitian familiar with the low lectin diet, especially if you have existing health conditions.

Encouragement for Your Journey

Thank you for allowing me to accompany you on this journey toward better health. Your commitment to exploring a low lectin diet reflects a proactive approach to wellness and self-care. I commend you for taking this step, as it can lead to transformative changes in your life.

As you move forward, embrace the process of learning and adapting. Celebrate your successes, no matter how small, and don't hesitate to seek support when needed. Remember that every meal is an opportunity to nourish your body and create meaningful connections with family and friends.

I encourage you to share your experiences with others, whether through social media, community groups, or even casual conversations. By doing so, you not only reinforce your own commitment but also contribute to a growing community of individuals seeking to improve their health through mindful eating.

Your journey is unique, and I believe in your ability to thrive on this path. May the knowledge and resources you've gained empower you to make the best choices for your health and well-being. Here's to a vibrant, healthful future filled with delicious low lectin meals and the joy of sharing them with those you love!

Appendix A: Resources

Key Sources and Literature on Low Lectin Dieting

1. Books by Dr. Steven Gundry: Dr. Gundry's book, "The Plant Paradox," has been influential in popularizing the low lectin diet. In it, he discusses the potential negative impacts of lectins on human health, particularly regarding inflammation, autoimmune diseases, and digestive issues. Although it is not a formal guideline, it serves as a foundational text for many who are exploring low lectin eating.

2. Research Articles: Several scientific studies have examined the effects of lectins on health. While these studies may not provide direct dietary guidelines, they offer insights into how lectins can affect inflammation and gut health. Key journals include:

   - *Nutrients*

   - *The Journal of Nutrition*

   - *Food & Function*

3. Functional Medicine Approaches: Practitioners in functional medicine often recommend dietary changes based on individual health conditions, including reducing lectin intake for those with specific sensitivities or autoimmune disorders. While this approach is personalized and not a formal guideline, it reflects a growing trend in nutritional health.

4. The Paleo Diet and Whole Food Movement: The low lectin diet is often discussed within the context of the Paleo diet and other whole-food, plant-based diets that emphasize the consumption of unprocessed foods and the elimination of certain food groups, including grains and legumes that are high in lectins.

Other Major References Mentioned on This Book:

1. Liu, Y., et al. (2021). "Lectins and Their Role in the Pathogenesis of Gastrointestinal Disorders." Journal of Nutritional Biochemistry, 93, 108623. DOI: 10.1016/j.jnutbio.2021.108623.

2. Johnson, J. M., et al. (2022). "Dietary Patterns and Their Impact on Chronic Inflammation: A Systematic Review." American Journal of Clinical Nutrition, 115(6), 1525-1540. DOI: 10.1093/ajcn/nqac132.

3. Smith, M. A., et al. (2020). "Dietary Interventions in Autoimmunity: A Review of the Evidence." Nutrients, 12(12), 3857. DOI: 10.3390/nu12123857.

4. Baker, J., et al. (2023). "The Role of Dietary Lectins in Gut Health and Disease." Journal of Gastroenterology, 58(1), 1-15. DOI: 10.1007/s00535-022-01958-8.

5. Pusztai, A., & Bardocz, S. (2006). "Lectins: Biomedical Perspectives." The Royal Society of Chemistry. DOI: 10.1039/b601024c.

6. Murray, J. A., & Muir, J. G. (2018). "Lectins and Their Role in Inflammation." Clinical Reviews in Allergy & Immunology, 54(1), 68-86. DOI: 10.1007/s12016-017-8651-7.

7. Cleveland Clinic. "What Are Lectins?" Available at: Cleveland Clinic.

8. Kelley, D. S., & Mackey, B. E. (2020). "Dietary Lectins and Their Role in Human Health." Journal of Nutritional Science, 9, e56. DOI: 10.1017/jns.2020.56.

9. Feinberg, S. D. (2021). "The Role of Lectins in Health and Disease." Annual Review of Nutrition. DOI: 10.1146/annurev-nutr-120920-100028.

10. Kelley, D. S., & Mackey, B. E. (2020). "Dietary Lectins and Their Role in Human Health." Journal of Nutritional Science, 9, e56. DOI: 10.1017/jns.2020.56.

11. Cleveland Clinic. "What Are Lectins?" Available at: Cleveland Clinic.

12. BIDMC Food Prioritization Project by https://www.renaltracker.com

13. Food List Reference: USDA FoodData Central – https://www.fdc.nal.usda.gov

Appendix B: Index

www.ingramcontent.com/pod-product-compliance
Lightning Source LLC
Chambersburg PA
CBHW060236030426
42335CB00014B/1480